Murphy Didn't Know: A Second Look

Kristin Blizzard

Presented by Blizzard Publishing

Kristin Blizzard

What Murphy Didn't
Know: A Second Look

Murphy Didn't Know: A Second Look

First printing
Made in the USA

Blizzard Publishing
978-1-387-02285-4

Kristin Blizzard

Find love for one another, forgive yourself for your past, believe in yourself, and most importantly have the tenacity to get up when you fall... this is how the ones that love you the most already see you!

Murphy Didn't Know: A Second Look

Kristin Blizzard

First, I want to thank my father and Trish for their love and support. My cousin Karen has always been there. I thank my brother, Shane. Bryan my better half. My second family Jaton, Gary T, Jill and Mini-Jill, Francine, Lori, Laura (Thank you so much). My Ohio family, Jamie, Wayne, and lil man. Debi, Wendy, Amy, Tony, Dr. K, Jackie, Bec, Bernie, Ellen, Susie, Pat, Marietta, James, BJ and Kylee. My buddy who kept everything safe for me, James, Gloria, Anne, and Andrea. My sisters Steph, Margo, Barb and our brother Robert.

Murphy Didn't Know: A Second Look

From the day four strikes of thunder were delivered onto this Earth by the tainted hand of man, we as a society have given into terror and fear. We have fought those and never learned anyone can kill with a weapon but not everyone is strong enough to live on. I am not debating Darwin's Theory of Evolution; I am merely referencing the evolution of mankind. There are facts that are infallible. There have been physical features particular to the plant, animal, or bird that have evolved. We must look for the changes to the mind. Life is more complicated now so we need find what makes us happy.

Every living has it's pros and cons, yet one must decide how precious the life is. Years after the steel bent, we agree to use that moment to define a generation. We may have bared our souls, but we did not falter. It is in every nation, every soldier, every child, every father and every mother that steps from this time that will set up what is to happen next. The world together celebrates tragedies and well as those events that lift us. An example is that twelve years before 9/11, in 1989 the wall did come down separating Germany. Again, in this world people rose up and stood for the freedom of a country.

We cannot erase fear and replace it with free will if their fears have our finger prints. Of course, humans are not perfect and sometimes terrible things happen. Socialization is not simply black and white. There will always be a grey. I find another word that more accurately defines the grey: perception.

Mankind has survived thus far by not isolating people, rather we continue building and evolving into a society in hopes for a peaceful surrender. We help one another and slowly we are finding more in common. In today's age, we are a smarter people because we have allowed ourselves to embrace and display equality. There is a repetition in stories of goodness, a blind kindness. This is our time and our thoughts. They often say, "The sins of the father are the sins of the son". We are a vast society that is made of so many

Murphy Didn't Know: A Second Look

generations. If are to continue recreate the blame then we will allow the stigma to lead us.

We are creating a better world. Old stigmas have been over overcome and equality displays strength and new hope. Wealth distributed slowly, moving as quality is becoming more important than the everyday. Good and bad are tossed around as the World Wide Web gives everyone a voice. Some even use it to help others show those cute kitten and puppy pics. I just have to point the fact I linked a better world with cute animal pics, (I believe a first). We witness the struggles, pain, and the even passing. We may not all understand, in the small bits of time, no one person will be changing the times. It will require the vast majority looking to create this. All of us working exchanging together to in fact bring people together. We are sociable species yet we are also a jealous one as well.

As money moves hands, it is easy to get lost in the moment. Once we begin to have money we forget those that put us in that position. Also, remember and embrace those that helped and forgive but always keep the face of those whom have opposed you. Otherwise, there is no doubt that we may lose the opportunity for growth. Our prejudices aside, we must find the common bond that links us as humans before the distinctions of what differences the nations becomes that of global extinction.

too often lacking the depths we once possessed. This is the time for us all to Murphy's Law clearly states the belief of what can go wrong will most certainly go wrong. We use this pessimistic approach to find humor when circumstances are not as we would prefer. Perhaps there are other ways to look at life; even in jest this concept applies a negative aura to our everyday lives. Instead of allowing the possibility for everything to be wrong, we must look to find comfort in everything that is right. Murphy might have not known, yet I have found anyone that knew everything. There is a beautiful surprise that lies inside blunders, it reminds of human error. That links all of us so try to things in stride.

Our past is filled with heroes both from life and pen. We create martyrs that verify our need to find acceptance in every situation. There comes a time when the understanding of one another means we will first have to find and understand ourselves. There is a simple goodness in everyone, have we forgotten the basics which means actually recognizing the good in others becomes an emotional not a rational thought. We must accept within every human is both good and bad. We can only encourage either.

Even as we can feel the warmth of others we are get back our own lives and regain the hope we had once lost. Hope is more than a sign we hold up when anguish is confronted. We find hope by living each day as opportunity and each person as human. We do this by opening the line of communication and looking at ourselves and holding ourselves responsible for the actions we take and the decisions we make.

We assume other's differences as failures. We all posse a greatness, as the "common man" shows the value and greatness of the overall society. Truly no one can be common if they live their life to their own potential. We all must judge only our own actions and thought. When we label others as immoral, we assume we know what is in the hearts of others. Is this not the new prejudices that formulate into hate? We are so quick to judge what others may do, if we see them as different we find ourselves feeling threatened. Our perception is what needs to be adjusted. We have learned history does indeed point to what our future may hold. We need to take notes and see the early warning signs. Perhaps there is a better world for all of us if we can learn to believe in ourselves and support the values and opinions of others.

Life does not have to be a guessing game but it is truly a people game. Today we must find ways for peace, find love for not just others but ourselves is a wonderful way to start us on our journey.

Murphy Didn't Know: A Second Look

Law #1 - It amazes me how the everyday simplicities can determine the basis of who we are and hold so much truth as to what it is that defines us as individuals. Using this as a basis for mutual respect, we look unto the ageless wisdom; "Do onto others as you would have them done unto you."

This is nothing short of the poetic notion of ebullience freeing itself from its deepest roots to blossom and grow into goodness toward our fellow mankind. We should all demand this from ourselves and one another. Why would we choose to accept a lesser person with lesser capabilities? Striving to excel as a person, we have the right to choose people that make a positive change within our own lives and values.

.

In a mere moment, we alter fate by how we treat one another. As we brutalize our values, we stand against one another. It takes just a moment to sit back and debate if we are doing right by ourselves and those around us? Are we as kind to others as we see ourselves being? If you are unsure whether your actions and words are doing wrong to another, just ask yourself but only one question. "Am I treating others the same way that I would like to be treated?" If you do not get a yes, then perhaps you may want to consider taking a step back and evaluate the situation. We are all responsible for each other just as we are all responsible for ourselves.

We are all human destined to have errors, on the other side we do have the ability to forgive. We need to once and for all stop telling our children one thing and do another. Be that person you are hoping others will be to you.

Law #2 - William Shakespeare cornered age-old wisdom when his epic masterpiece personified self-realization the moment he saw he could never be true to anyone else without first being true to himself. We can cast a thousand walls to keep others out, or perhaps we may use these same walls to barricade our true self inside. Either way from the stroke of a pen to paper set in motion for generations yet to come the reality is we can never be honest with others if we do not see the truth within ourselves. Once this metamorphosis happens, you have the potential the transformation will take you and nourish you, so you may blossom into all that is good and precious? The entire ordeal of ever even needing to change is chalked up to another life altering personal victory. The sacred prize of knowing who you are and it is the first step to who you may become.

Law #3 - When we take into consideration exactly how much time we have on this Earth and the number of people we will encounter, we all must

Murphy Didn't Know: A Second Look

look at how will we effect other's lives and how will they affect our own. Simply breaking down the actual time we do have per person shows how precious very minute is. It is a simple fact there will never be enough time to celebrate the good. Unfortunately, how many of us focus on that precious good? Most of us dwell on the mediocrity. We see our pains of yesterday, concerns for today and our fear of what tomorrow will cast. The negative cloud loom's around us destroying the positive that everyone is entitled to find. It is difficult to feel chronic pain and find joy for the future. We can understand the pain only gets worse and our spirits only damper. Perhaps it would be wiser to embrace each other in times of good and bad. I would rather love endless then to love safely. The reality is that the times of grandeur speeches enticing society to evolve and grow together are gone. The newer generations have much kinder hearts and do champion for equality for the most part. Endless negative chatter must stop. I hope when the opportunity arrives, we allow our hearts to govern the mind rather than the mind dictating what the heart is permitted to feel. Perhaps when chance brings by a new face, you realize that your time with this person is a blessing and you run with that goodness and pursue it with vengeance.

Kristin Blizzard

I can say the people in my life are kind and genuine rather than rude and hateful; they all have encouraged me to write. I would like to see people enjoying the lives even more. I want to expose those that are wicked and let those wonderful people I am blessed to have in my life known they are appreciated and loved.

Law #4 - An almost punishable sense for fairness of all situations may seem lucent to the ideal humanist, but the victory is reached when it is used to repeal actions and in some cases inaction against injustices. Many people feel an internal conflict to insure right always conquers all inequalities. Often one hears about righteousness but how often do we see the actions and positively reinforce the kindness from others. This can begin just one person trying to carry righteousness as a calling may serve as an example for others to follow. People for the most part want to be good. Most of us would rather show that positive glow. Perhaps others may follow suit and look into themselves for a similar calling. One person should not hold the entire burden, nor is there one person that is capable of the duty. However; it may only take one to inspire others to share in the positive connection we usually keep only for those closest to us. It is very exhausting to try to live this life. Instead of fighting every injustice we come across, it may make a bit more sense to choose which battles are

Murphy Didn't Know: A Second Look

actually worth fighting. The concept of a perfect world is beautiful in thought and is quite desirable; however, it is also very impractical. There is nothing wrong with being a noble person; after all, we do try to teach our children to be good to others. Somehow when the age of 18 is crossed our society accepts less. Children are held to a higher level. I might suggest we retrain the "adult thinking and priorities." The greatest asset is hope. We should have hope with one another and trust others will have hope in us. Doing the right thing is normally not the easy thing, but I would remind you before you make any decision you must decide if your action represents what you have lived your entire life. It has taken many arguments and yet, still for many they have not realized, words do not change a society: hope does.

Law #5 - I you desire change in any form, then find the options and contemplate. How many people agree with your findings? The power of the people can change everything.

Presently, I hear a majority of people seek change in the government. Let your congress know. You hire these people via your vote. If you lose because of policy job, they will lose their jobs. The people in office should represent your beliefs. Refusing to vote on a bill for 8 months. Find out if your boss would get happy to pay you when you fail to do your job.

Law #6 - Perception is everything! Reality is at best one's perception. We all may see one entity; however, the perception of the image may vary from one to another. Personal life experiences, culture, prejudices, fears, thoughts, ECT… all change our views. Even if what someone is searching for is staring them in the face, if they do not see it, then it does not exist for them.
What is right for one person may not be right for the next one to come along! I only have the right to decide what is acceptable for me. I hope that most have a similar concept so the tint of their reality is close enough to my own that we may realize a similar reality. Regardless to my own thoughts, I do have to respect other opinions and I can choose to take or not take them into consideration. Some people do see a completely different reality and no one has the right to figure the value and worth of someone else's thoughts.

Law #7 - Money has some awesome powers; it has the power to tempt when temptation may not have been there. We can move a mountain, swim across an ocean, or even fly through the skies. Just as it may feed a million hungry faces, it can also lead people down a horrid path. Money is most powerful when we allow it to corrupt who we are.

Murphy Didn't Know: A Second Look

So many great things can be accomplished with the aid of funds, but it is never the money that does the good deeds, I am sure if one was to look beyond that all mighty green, there would be a person or people that should maybe get the acknowledgement, even if they choose to not accept it.

Law #8 - To the uninspired, a dream is a distant mirage. To so many dreams are simply unattainable and it is best to focus on the goals already set into motion. If one believes in themselves, anything can happen. If you just have faith in yourself and are willing to put the time and effort into whatever it is you desire to accomplish, then that mirage has become a goal. The only difference between a goal and a dream is in the goal you have some ideas on how to make it come true, a dream needs but a path mapped out. Instead of allowing your dreams to fall, why not spend the time attempting to figure which is the road you need to take. Everyone has the chance to live as they desire, but are all too often quieted by those that bring them down, often even before they have even started. Once you do throw in the towel on either a dream or a goal, neither will have a possibility to come true; then they both will remain a fantastic mirage

Law #9 - It is with a softened heart we find laughter and the gift to hopefully share that humor. I do advise though to be quite cautious when your laughter is at the expense of others. You never know when the chance of luck twisting against your run of fortune, and then you find that those jokes were maybe not so nice to others. It is pretty much a sure thing to say no matter how amusing you find yourself or your material, the probability of your humor interfering with someone else's happiness is a rather high probability. There is humor in irony and many people do have common threads that do bear humor, however, there is normally one person that is going to take the joke a bit far. The human spirit is the one thing I believe should never find ridicule.

When we open the door to the human spirit, we open the door for other to do the same. As nice as it to share the gift of laughter, it is a true gift if there are no feelings hurt and most importantly no one feels the salt in their wounds to make others laugh. After all, if you have to hurt others to get a laugh, how funny are you anyway?

Law #10 - Many of the general population strives to become a bit more successful, maybe a little more powerful, and even maybe to have a few more friends. With what you would like to better yourself in, please know nothing you can ever achieve, own, or know is more imperative then the self-respect you have. Who you hope to become in the future is the greatest decision you will ever make. If you decide to sell out, then you not only sellout who you are but also your future. Not only are you stuck with losing yourself, but how about those empathetic eyes never knowing who you really were. For all you know you were once destined to inspire a new world of hope and prosper but with an uncontrollable thirst, you no longer are that person that was given the privilege to inspire hope. The one thing to remember with whatever you decide to do, you have until you draw your last breath to change so there is never a too late unless you never make the effort.

Law #11 - Life is a gift so why not live it! It is so tempting to allow yourself to give into the guilt and dismay from our own actions. Once you have made amends with that negative emotion we all keep inside, let it go. Everyone does make mistakes and we sometimes are much too hard on ourselves. That time would be much better spent making things right rather than dwelling in the past. Once you do let go of those emotions you do allow yourself to begin mending a broken heart. I am sure it is safe to say everyone does have a piece of a broken heart trying to mend somewhere. When it comes to the pain others have hurt us with, we normally figure in and accept the blame and guilt. Again, the guilt and blame is not what is needed: time, love, care, gentleness, and understanding are the ingredients to get past those memories and thoughts. Once you clear out all of that negativity, you have room for the good stuff, and I do promise you will find more room in your heart for the good then you have for the bad.

Law #12 - Nourishing the mind begins with nourishing the body. Eating well, sleeping well, a proper diet, and an adequate amount of daily exercise are all very necessary ingredients to the improvement of and maintaining your overall health. I can assure you I am not pushing any diet or marathon to anyone any time soon. I do believe you should contact your doctor before making any significant changes to your life style. On the other hand, I am suggesting the little things we can all do to help is where we need to start. We do spend more time on focusing on our bodies and forget that our minds need care too. Perhaps a little daily reflection would not be a bad decision and actually quite helpful. It is the same with the body; I see nothing wrong with enjoying a glass of wine or maybe a bite of chocolate. Just stay within balance of what is good and what is good for you. Having a healthier body and mind are the rewards. It is not a one-time thing; it does take commitment, time, energy, and when it's a little tough, you might even need to get a little help. It is a lot of work to abide by a healthy lifestyle. if you have never follow e done, but you are so worth it. Everyone deserves to feel good, this just happens to be something you might be able to control.

Law #13 - As tough and cruel as others can be, when things are at their toughest, when you are thinking the world has taken over and you have nothing to hold on to, all I can say is for you to find comfort in your faith. I do believe faith can exist and whether you attach a religion to it or not, perhaps you have faith in humankind, or perhaps you have faith in yourself. I believe if one chooses to believe in any religion that is their personal choice and how they devote themselves to whatever they decide is not something anyone else or I have the right to question. To simplify it, this is a crazy world and the trials and obstacles are going to be out there for us all to overcome, and everyone does run across the day that the burdens pile up and it feels like the whole world is caving in. Have faith in yourself and others, this is the key to finding peace within every situation. Everyone does have someone or something out there for better or worse, and often as the times seem too hectic you might not see the hands above you trying to help you get out of the situation. Just because you have been blinded to their existence, does not take them away, perhaps if you were out of the proverbial box you would see what is truly around you. The fact none of us are alone I hope gives you a reason to keep going.

Law #14 - We have all heard the masterfully composed speech striking and courageous, "We have nothing to fear but fear itself". Fear have to be one of the harshest four-letter words in the English language, it sends shivers down the spine and freezes the night until we keep our selves awake in this decay known as insecurities. Fear itself is a wonderful gift we all have. It is a very raw animal instinct and the fact we have an internal warning system so we can recognize a possible bad situation is not fate insuring the worst is to come. Instead of seeing it as a time to run, it would be best to be used as a caution and a good time to evaluate your current course of action. We should embrace and use fear to its potential. We never should be overrun by our fear; we can use it to navigate us through any possible troubles ahead. Using it may be just what you need to get through situations, perhaps you need to slow down on your present course or you may need to take an alternate route. Mother Nature has given us all the ability to know when things may be hazardous or something good or bad may happen. Maybe we do not have the ability to alter our fate, but we can ensure or lessen what is to come.

Law #15 - Love is beautiful, love is grandeur, love is a very graceful emotion that carries with it a burning passion if lit can explode into everything we can and do desire. We sometimes do look at love and let a blinded rage or furry itself and manifests itself into a righteous fearless conqueror and whether the reality it is worthy, the raw emotion has swept away and battles are fought. Whether they were necessary is irrelevant and before anyone has time to view the situation the damage has already been done. Love is worth fighting for at times; I am sometimes quite impractical and become blinded during some situations. I have learned quite the lessons and it is good to insure what you are fighting over warrants and even more importantly agrees in your actions. There are times when the fist is the weakest force and perhaps the pen or even sweet whispered words are the much more powerful and deliver the needed blow. There are times when we must wager a war and when that time comes, I hope everyone does see what is at stake. When the need confronts you to a stand up against your adversary please take in consideration they feel as strong as you and both of you are people filled with emotions, and it is much easier to inflict injury upon others if it is in the name of love. I believe only when you have no other option, you have attempted all other resources, then, and only then do you raise arms to anyone. I am also quite impulsive and follow my heart more often than my head. I do hope what you are fighting for is worth what is left in the end after the fighting ceases and reflection does not turn you away or you love away from you.

Law #16 - With all societies merging to form one massive global society, the age of primal attacks theoretically would have found its end. We attempt to save the rain forest, save the whales, and even save the Earth; however, we accept a cycle of genocide as we punish the generation before, we build hate that filters down to the next generations. Until the wounds heal, an endless cycle builds up velocity until it is aimed and set forth into motion. Many philosophers have concurred with each other's findings; we as the human race are likely to find extinction by our own doings. Knowing most people are good does not stop the concern. As a global society, perhaps we may intervene and replace the hate with love, the rage with compassion, and the foreseen with promise of tomorrow. The glory of today is finding the peace within knowing that yesterday has been forgiven and tomorrow is still full with possibilities.

Murphy Didn't Know: A Second Look

Law #17 - The most prized possessions are always the ones we have earned. In matters of personal natures just as in business, there are sometimes monetary values attached to the finish line. What you have earned surpasses the ribbons or trophies on the wall! Not everyone has the courage to try from the beginning, so simply joining the race you already have achieved success.

Law #18 - Please know, as the times may seem to get rough and everyday struggles tend to push your limits, it is still is your life. For good or bad, your destiny lays in your hands. There is never the right day to wish your life away. The times may lead you to believe you passed the time of desperation. In the eve of internal destruction approaches and you bow your head to your solemn upcoming demise please stop right there. Temptation may point toward this as a last resort as you may feel as if you have exhausted all other options; but there is always another route. I know some people have the gift to know how glorious and fantastic life may be, but no one has the perfect life. As humans, we are all very vulnerable and I have found from personal experience that those that gloat the most usually hurt the most. Innocent comments can rip apart the tormented and no- one is ever the wiser. The first step is to realize there is a problem and you need to get some help. There are always people out there that want to help others they just do not know where to find the people needing help. Please if you ever think you have passed the line of ever coming back, you go get help immediately. Go to a local emergency room or there are numbers to call to get help right away. You never have to bear this alone; there is always a hand out trying to reach you. All you have to do is reach out to them, and then together you can tackle the demons and find peace. You may never have the spoils others enjoy; however, you are very likely to be the most valuable spoil to someone.

Law #19 - You should always be proud of who you are. In the end, we must not look at what we were able to gather, rather what we did with what we had. If life were only about what we can attain, we would call it monopoly instead of life. Typically, people are graded on a social scale by the possessions they display. Any one person can find the ability to gain riches and survey from atop of a mountain, but then they would be a spectator and miss the opportunity to compete in life. Rather than attempting to weigh any economical or structured value why not try some self-reflection. I would rather be the one that tried to help a million people then to have held a million dollars.

Murphy Didn't Know: A Second Look

Law #20 - Following the last concept, laughter is an excellent tool and gift to be shared by everyone including you. If you have something to share with others that would brighten another's day then please shine away.

Law #21 - As we all know, the "perfect family" is just an urban legend. The family you are born into is one factor you can never change. I hope that you can see past the DNA line when determining who family is and who isn't. It is a travesty to limit those to whom you choose to love by simply discarding the possibilities based not on their merit, but by negating them based on heredity. No one can choose where he or she is from; they can only decide where they go from here on.

Law #22 - As children grow, we hope their parents do guide them down the path of goodness and knowing right from wrong. We teach them and mold them in the earlier stages of life to our own ideal and morals. Peers do have a strong force and are the source of most parents' nightmares. Often in the early preteen years through the later teen years, peers have more control over our kids then we do. It brings little consonance during those trying times whether a child will stand up and yield to their conscience depends on the seeds planted in the early days. After they have had an explanation of the consequences and facts, all anyone can do is to hope the guidance you have given them along with their own sense of fairness will playout and they will choose the right thing.

Law #23 - Being a good person is hopefully something you want to do because of who you are not because of whom someone else is. It is very admirable to want to show others the respect they deserve; however, it is more admirable respecting others because you desire the same respect for yourself. I am simply stating you should be good and respectful to others not for whom they may or may not be, rather be that person because it is a testament to how wonderful you are.

Law #24 - In case you are unaware of the origin of the word goodbye, it has been shortened from May God be with you or go with God. This may have you rethink idea of wishing your loved ones away. This does comes from a time even more uncertain then our own presently.

Law #25 - Life mimics that little sticker in your rear- view mirror, objects are closer then what may appear. Sometimes we are all too close to the situation to realize something good or bad is about to happen. Everyone needs to take a moment out of

Murphy Didn't Know: A Second Look

a busy day and to look for what is happening in the world around him or her. The strangest times are when we do not look for anything in particular to happen, we have no expectations, and suddenly we are living in a foreign world. Perhaps it is a good idea to take some time for yourself, go find some birds to sing to you, or maybe go outside and let the sun warm your face.

Law #26 - It is wonderful to see your cultural background and to embrace it. Color of one's skin has nothing to do with how rich in culture a society is. If you truly believe the color of one skin decides the importance of another person or whether they are a gift to the rest of the world. The world is in color. The world has greens, pinks, blues, oranges, and even more. If you are stuck in the black and white then you my friend lose.

Law #27 - I know the oldest question is why are we all here, what is our purpose if any? Just because we may not know exactly why does not lessen the importance of people. Some may be have a longer stay on this earth and some are gone before they ever even open their eyes. Who are any of us to decide the value of the miracle or how significant they are? You may have been here for more than a hundred years and still not know your purpose, but then perhaps those hundred years are your purpose; maybe that is why you were place here. The all mighty question still remains unanswered: even now, no one can figure it out. There is nothing wrong with living your life today with goodness we all share, then as those final moments appear, allow your fate to decide if you have fulfilled the reasons of why.

Law #28 - The promise of tomorrow begins with accepting the faults of yesterday and trying not to repeat them today. If you can learn the lesson the first time and educate the next generation of our mistakes then we may have the capability of preventing the same situation from resurfacing. No one has the power to know what will happen in the future for certain, so it is worth our every effort and we must use all lessons the past has given us to prevent the disasters of humanity from ever happening again. If there is nothing else that comes with the sorrow brought from our own actions, would to prevent the same tears to spread into whatever the future holds for us.

Law #29 - The beautiful act of forgiving has nothing to do with agreeing or defending a situation. Forgiving is the first step to find inner peace with what happened to move on and not allowing yourself to become a victim twice. When you become enslaved to the darkness in your mind then the incident has not ended, and every day you fall as the pain eats you alive. Once you are able to forgive the situation, the nightmares end and then your life belongs to you again.

Law #30 - Applying justice is nothing more then awarding or punishing according to a set standard of law or order. One person is never the deciding vote, in all forms of government, it takes the majority to form one principle and establish what is necessary to maintain these guidelines. Right and wrong should always be the deciding factor for the outcome that is more suitable for the offence given the exact circumstances, not a temperament full of anger and loathing. Justice normally will never completely make up what has happened for the victim or their family. Some losses can never really find the justice they deserve to replace what has been taken away. It is never fair when a jury can decide the fate of someone whom by no fault of their own must depend on people they have never met to recognize and punish those whom are at fault. Civil actions are a perfect example, when someone's life is altered permanently, how can any sum of money replace the lifestyle and security they enjoyed before the incident happened? Some people believe the sum awarded should have limits, but then I ask you, how much are your loved ones worth to you?

Law #31 - Responsibility is the defining measure of a productive adult. Mistakes are part of being human. Acting responsibly is making the best decision in sight and carrying it out. Everyone is going to mess something thing up, it is ok, fix it to the best of your capabilities and then you can move on. With age just comes a few more years of opportunity to learn the difference between right and wrong. There are many sixteen-year old's with more common sense then some fifty-year old's.

Law #32 - With every person you meet, you have an obligation to facilitate a guided communication with them to the best of your abilities. Reach out with a bit of Spanglish, perhaps bake a bunch of cookies for the neighbors, even wine make a great gift to a new neighbor. We are not limited by only our words, arts, and culture; we all have the ability to cross over and use others' words, arts, and culture. Personally, I do prefer articulated speech with a bit of humor. It is a sign of creativity, intelligence, and culture. Some people for whatever reason do not have the ability to speak but may have a lot to add. It is everyone's reasonability to reach out to them and lend them our voices to share their words, everyone has something they

Murphy Didn't Know: A Second Look

can contribute, sometimes we need to reach out to them and listen to what they have inside.

Law #33 - It does not matter if you work from 9-5 or 5-9, whenever do work, you should know by now, there is life outside of work. I understand many people are so passionate about whatever the work is that they do, even in the off time people might get together and even then, everyone talks about work. We want to work hard to improve our overall quality of life, but pleased not take this too far. Everyone and it does not matter if you are the CEO of a major corporation or a cashier at a local gas station; everyone needs to take some time and look at their reasons for working so hard. It is so easy to be caught up in working hard for that one day when life is just a bit sweeter just realize you may notice one day it has already passed you by. Bees are born to work, we are people, and we are born to live. In a perfect world, everyone can take off two weeks a year and head out to the vacation of a lifetime every year. The reality is many have to work every day to earn that paycheck so they do not fall behind. Even if you have but 1 hour a day or even a week, take a moment and look into the reason you are pushing yourself so hard. Even if it is to provide a roof over your head, then take a moment to enjoy that roof.

Law #34 - Imagination is where all new ideas, concepts, and thoughts begin. It is when we pursue our imagination with questions, we begin to develop answers and use that creativity to improve upon everyday life. A great mind can envision change before it is developed and it takes an amazing mind to look beyond the average eye and apply that change into the next stage of development.

Law #35 - It is neither fun to be driving down the road or living life with no clue where you are. When the question of direction on the pavement it is rather difficult to figure it out, just look at a map or stop and ask. However; when you are on the road of life there are no maps to follow but there is a real ways people that would be happy to try to help you answer the same questions. If you think, you are lost, good chance you very well might be. Pull over and just ask for help, for myself, the more I just drive around the until more lost begins to look familiar.

Law #36 - An inspiration conforms to a mental awareness for the purpose of enlightenment. We compare the eccentric to the insane while the rest enjoy the serenity of fine a set standard. This concept has long past stayed its welcome. Find your muse and grow with it. You should strive for

Murphy Didn't Know: A Second Look

your muse to electrify you and heighten all of your senses. Leave the ordinary and look toward your passions, find that inspiration and allow your mind to be bound by no limits. Everyone deserves the chance to open their mind; you just need to worry less about what people are going to think. As long as you are not hurting anyone else in the process, then no one really has the right to interfere. One should never be defined or limited by the inabilities of others to see outside possibilities.

Law #37 - It is ok to see the beauty each one of us possess. Everyone has something different that does make them so amazingly beautiful and I do believe everyone out there does have that one person that was born to love them and to be with them. To them no one else exists. Please know you are both beautiful inside and on the outside. It is very common for people to glance into a mirror and see their doubts and fears rather than themselves. Maybe this is a great day for you to stop seeing what you do not like about yourself, and start focusing on what you do like. A mirror does show the truth; however, our perception is often tainted by what our mind may or may not see.

Kristin Blizzard

Law #38 - If you look at your daily routines as hectic and disorganized: perhaps you need to identify any obstacles and take some to set up a system that will accommodate you and your lifestyle. There are many tools available to help you organize and prioritize your daily routines. Just take a look at what your needs are and go from there.

Law #39 - From deep within the purest of all hearts lay every and anything one would need to find happiness. Love is the wind that lets us soar into the deepest roots of our own souls and find peace. I know the "romantics" read verses spelling out profound theory of untamed love burning into literary history. A love like this is benevolent to say the least; yet it is but only a small bit of the entire picture of love. It is common to get lost inside of the midst of the grandeur; however, love does have its hardships and trials. Love surpasses the common thread of humanity and allows for error and human nature's mistakes. Who believes if you love someone, then if circumstances forced separation, who would be so careless to let that love free to go? True love eradicates any preconceived lines drawn. To love another person endlessly, we must do what is best for them, not always what we may prefer to do. Their happiness is ultimately the concern. There are times when we must over look our own feelings and biased beliefs and let the one we love who they

Murphy Didn't Know: A Second Look

are meant to be. As much as anyone would want to make another person happy, sometimes things just are not meant to be, and as much as it hurts, if you holding on to something that is not yours to hold, it will hurt more in the end. The human spirit is never to be a prisoner to simply be suppressed against its will. If that time does come to play, then perhaps you may find peace knowing that you have memories that will only fade when you allow them to. For excellent reasons, historically love has been compared to the likeness of a rose. If you cultivate and allow the love to grow it will blossom, but at the same time, if you try to control the love, it can very easily tear into you. The more you fight it the more scars it will leave. The miracle of both the rose and love is how fragile and beautiful they are and yet both have a very tough exterior.

Law #40 - Why does it appear when you need time away from the world to figure life out; it seems as if the entire population has conspired to interfere by using all means necessary? Our greatest inventions are used to proficiently harass those whom we love the most and even prevent them from completing even the most obscure task.

Law #41 - Sometimes when the times are looking to be the worst it is the best time to sit back and laugh at the situation. We all have faced those times that getting through it seems to be an impossible task. That is when the timing is the best. How many people think about finding laughter to get through a situation? Instead of exploding into a deeper hole, it would be effort best spent on trying to set your mental health in good balance. Small problems are gigantic when ones you are not grounded.

Law #42 - The greatness of a relationship reveals the immeasurable about of love shared between the parties. It is amazing the characteristics we cherish most in ones we love are also the same nail biting flaws. Persistence becomes stubbornness just as sensitivity falls as weakness. An argument is a raging fire and the yelling is the smoke. Perhaps if we looked outside of the situation and realized why we care about the person we are angry with and voiced it, we would smother the fire out.

Law #43 - A very simple note to remember, no one can love more than they have the ability to. You may fall in love with someone that is unable to feel the same way as you. Often feelings get hurt when we pour ourselves into a relationship without the desired response. We all fall in love, for whatever reason, but just as we cannot change how people love us in return, we cannot just stop loving that person either. True love is unconditional. True love can weather any storm, any circumstance, or any doubt if given the chance. Facing the situation may still be very difficult, but it is a test of love for oneself as well as the love shared. Honesty can be quite painful as many are unable to face the truth. If there is ever is a truth needing to be exposed, you need to find the strength and courage and find comfort in knowing those that love you the most are the safest people to confide in. It is a test of a faith in all relationships and those whom ride out the storm with you are the ones youkan count on. If there are differences either of you cannot see past, perhaps it is best to realize you need to end the relationship or alter your definition of the relationship.

Law # 44 - Typically, the best solution to any problem does not include violence. Anyone claiming differently either has known nothing else or has never truly witnessed its devastation.

Law # 45 - In the circle of life, there comes a time for everyone to face judgment. Whether there is an afterlife once we leave this world or not, every decision, every word, and every action throughout the span of your life defines what your life has meant. Often, we over look how we have treated others due to our beliefs and not on the merit of the other person. We look down on people for how they dress, how much money they have, or how they decide to live their life. To be an individual means you are different from others, and others are going to be different from you. It is easy to judge other lives when you are not the one that should atone and make retribution. Everyone has judged others at one point; however, we can hope that we become better as people and perhaps the next time the same situation arises we can look past our fears and accept others as we would like them to accept us. From the differences in all of us, either instinct or learned, others can see us beyond our present scope. You are responsible for yourself and for your fellow mankind. Some choices others make, may make you feel uncomfortable, but is it them or your own insecurities that create that need to downcast others?

Law #46 - The human mind is an amazing complex unit with unknown potential. Wisdom is priceless; when one considers all that may be accomplished with a little "know-how," we can see new opportunities begin to show up. As long as our minds wonder, we will continue to figure new thoughts into play. As long as there is someone wanting to know how something works, there will always be someone else willing to teach. This ageless cycle continues as new knowledge is blended with the old beliefs with hopes of bettering the world we live in. This has worked from the beginning of time, why would you think it would be different now?

Law #47 - We all have some skeletons left hanging in the old proverbial closet. Regret is merely time wasted on dwelling on past unchangeable aspects of your life. If we all spent less time on grieving for the past and more on preventing the past repeating itself, there would be less to grieve in the end. I have done many things I should not have, but what is important is I make the attempt to never repeat my mistakes. I have asked for forgiveness and tried to make amends when possible. Realistically thinking, what else is there for one to do after they have made amends?

Law #48 - The concept of controlling others' thoughts in any aspect is obtuse in a modern world. Even in times of physical restraints, the mind still is free to wonder. When we attempt to limit what another person may think, we limit their potential for not only themselves but also what they may have added to our society.

Law #49 - A race rewards is more abundant then any trophy can ever note. Sometimes we enter a race with ambitions deeper than the quest for first place. There is glory in effort regardless of ranking.

Kristin Blizzard

No one enters a race with the express intent of falling short of the finish line, but who to say simply getting back up after falling may not be the reward in the end? In the true spirit of competition, there is a line of respect given to all those whom stand up to the fate awaiting them on the other side of the finish line.

Law #50 - Many of us have fears that we let prevent ourselves from succeeding; the thought of greatness is deemed impossible. With every effort, it remains right out of our reach. Perhaps we have lost the understanding of greatness, but then again, perhaps we attach too much to the persona. Greatness is in the little things we all do every day; it is doing one good thing at a time with nothing less than the best intent whether it succeeds or not. We all need to believe in the goodness in people beginning with believing in ourselves. Anyone can write people off that fail short of our expectations but there will come a day when people will follow their own path whether they have other's approval or not. They too may be on their destined path of greatness.

Law #51 – If you see your community struggling, try volunteering. It will give you an opportunity to jump in and make the change you and hopefully start to end the struggling. Get involved!

Murphy Didn't Know: A Second Look

Law #52 - Any poet knows a poem is simply a thought transcending one concept into an expression. Shaping filth into radiance is never difficult if you use the surrounding beauty to open up the darkness. All cultures place a different emphasis on different areas relating to life; however, there is not aright one or a wrong one. They are just different. Culture is biased depending on the popular influences surrounding it. Most artists stray from the mainstream leaving them open to criticism. To educate oneself and appreciate the many forms or expression is the first step in understanding what attributes one possesses. Thus, the appreciation for other distinct cultures stems from a basic understanding of our own.

Law #53 - As the days pass by, I realize time is drifting away so easily. Slowly first the minutes fly by, then the hours seem to spin away. It is as if time is only important when it comes off a calendar. For some reason, we overlook our greatest gifts until they have been stripped from us. Why is it we do not appreciate or even notice what is in our life until we no longer have it in grasp? Those precious seconds we surrendered before are seconds of our life we can never get back. Instead of regretting the loss, it would be better energy and time better spent on cherishing the time we have left.

Kristin Blizzard

Law #54 - Just so you know that saying about making sure if you are ever in an accident to have clean underwear on is a crock! I assure you the underwear being clean makes little different. Just to clarify the subject, we shower and wear clean underwear because we want someone to care if we are in the accident.

Law #55 - In the shadows of a struggle we often hear the whispers (or shouts in some cases) of doubt. No matter how hard we try, we can never seem to stop those drowning voices. There comes a time when you need to stop listening to others and find the strength inside to do your own thing. Always listen to the voice of reason, but remember having faults are part of being human. No one is perfect; knowing this we can see what defines us and what it is we need to fight for and to hold on to, in order to become an individual.

Law #56 - In the midst of any ghastly storm lays an opportunity for some good to be found within the terror. There is always a positive lesson in the end of every day. Using this theory, much of everyday stress can be lifted from your shoulders. As long as you can find some good in every situation, there will always be a reason to continue trying.

Murphy Didn't Know: A Second Look

Law #57 - Youth is strength and experience is wisdom. If you locate where youth and experience meet, we hope justice is a common denominator of the two. As long as the youth have the energy to try to change things for the better and the experienced are wise enough to guide that power: we may not have to pass on mistakes of the previous generations. If any system no longer works for the benefit of its people then hopefully the vigor and wisdom serves as a means to establishing equality for all. It is amazing to watch as the times may change yet there are so many people refusing to change with them. Prejudices are never based on fairness. It is refreshing to know that the younger generations try to filter out the bigotry rather than the individuals.

Law #58 - The ebullience of gift giving is in the concept that there are people at any given time that are thinking of you. It releases the anxiety when circumstances prove to be going against you, there is someone out there thinking of you and willing to bet on you regardless of the circumstances.

Law #59 - There are so many reasons to want to befriend others. Some people do it for the right reasons and yet others whom have less noble reasoning. Some people may want to be your friend

Kristin Blizzard

for what you do for them, but as we all know, that really is not a good friend. Often after finding yourself with such "friends," the idea of never letting anyone close again seems to pop in to mind. The more people you do meet increases your chance in meeting others that will love you for who are inside, those will be the ones with you if bad fortune arises. They are the friends that will be there in the end; hopefully, those are the same friends you held on to through the many curves life throws at people.

Law #60 - As a society we all laugh and cry together whether it is from joy or tragedy. For the most part, we all have very similar hopes and dreams; and we are all plagued by similar fears. As we search out our differences as individuals, we show how similar we are. We all have rough times and may find ourselves struggling in those times. We all have good times even if they are far apart in between. No matter our similarities or differences, we are all here living this life given to each of us. The time for setting standards others are supposed to abide by are gone, now is the time we set our own standards, for ourselves.

Law #61 - I believe in mind of matter and I also do believe we should all look at everyday as an opportunity to do whatever you have set out to do.

Murphy Didn't Know: A Second Look

There are many obstacles in everyone's way. There is always a way to maneuver around any curve as long as the will to do so exists. A broken leg is a broken bone, and it may heal or it might not. It is something to overcome, not a wall. Each of us have obstacles, may they be physical or emotional. We all need to figure out what is holding us back, accept it, and then look for another path. Sometimes we may do this alone, other times we need a helping hand. Asking for help is far from swallowing pride, it is about realizing we are all humans and have the need for others. Either way we all need to realize the mind has always been stronger then the body, after all, it has convinced you to find doubt.

Law #62 - Some things in life are a bit more difficult to do than others. Putting a pair of jeans may not be hard for you. There are different ways to put them on. Most of us prefer the one leg at a time approach. If you jump in with both legs at once, you may run the risk of cracking your head on the floor. Life can be just like that old pair of jeans, sometimes it is best to take one day at a time and go from there.

Law #63 - There is no such thing as too many friends. It is fantastic to realize the roles they play in our daily happiness as well as the development of whom we will become. They are the ones that brighten our lives and maybe even teach us to lighten up sometimes.

Law #64 - Inside of this fast-paced society we live in today lies trash filled highways, polluted lakes and rivers, landfills over crowded, and of course the infested brown smog hovering over many cities. We have destroyed most of what Mother Nature has given to us. There must come a time we rebuild and replenish what has been taken. Instead of plowing down trees we could recycle more and use less while implementing the planting of new trees. Getting together with neighbors and friends to collect cans and bottles may go a long way in funding for improving playgrounds or restoring parks. Newton's law, "For every action there is a reaction," needs little clarifying. We need to invest in our environment before the damage cannot be reversed. A time will come when all of our resources have been depleted. We here today may not feel the impact, but look into your children's face and picture what we are leaving for them. If we do not find other resources, a day will come when society steps backwards.

Law #65 - You should never spend money you do not have. Do not count on it until it is in your hands. Banks do not care about hard luck stories. A problem for you is not necessarily a problem for them; you are liable for what you do. A bank's is a business. Their function is creating wealth for those that own the bank. In the long run, you will spend less if you stay within your means.

Law #66 - If you ever feel so stressed, like life is smothering your last breath from you, then maybe you need to find a place to relieve the tension. Here are a few thoughts for when you let things go: 1. Never scream in someone's ear (you will not win considerate points), 2. Do not physically or emotional take your anger out on someone else, 3. Do not hurt yourself! There is a lot of truth in the notion of exposing what is causing the pain does begin the healing process. It might hurt to get to the issue, but it is the only way to release what is causing the problem. There is nothing wrong with exhaling and releasing the bolted shut, pent up anger, just as it is not wise to further any wounds to yourself or anyone else.

Law #67 - When all is looking great and it appears nothing can go wrong: duck! Noting your life is well is very healthy. Believing nothing in this world can happen to ruin your day is begging for bad luck to visit. Please never stop enjoying the good because you are afraid of what might happen, just do not become arrogant and forget things can always be worse. Be happy for the good you have in your life now, enjoy the day as it is.

Law #68 - He whom picks his nose while driving must want to be pointed at and even ridiculed. There is not much worse than missing a traffic light because the guy in front of you refuses to move his fingers from his nose. We all at some point have the need sometimes to get rid of sinus troubles: there are ways to do so with class. Do not be frightened by the use of a tissue. I am referring to the habitual offenders.

Law #69 - As consumers, we all have a voice attached to the business we conduct. If you do not like the way a business chooses to conduct itself then stop patronizing them. It is senseless to accept less then you want. Where you go and what you do reflect the kind of person you are, so why go where your standards are not met. Many businesses have spent countless hours and money trying to create a customer friendly solution center. I like to give a business an opportunity to fix the problem. If they do not satisfy my needs as a consumer, they no longer will get my business. Economics teaches us the simple principle of supply and demand, which establishes completion. There are some excellent companies and those are the ones that get the repeat business. Your business comes from your

Murphy Didn't Know: A Second Look

hard-earned money and you should get what you pay for.

Law #70 - The invention and introduction of the television has altered the fiber of our society. We all have laughed and cried with our favorite characters even if it is those precious thirty minutes once a week. Many question if TV is a prodigy of society or if society is the prodigy of the TV. Perhaps they are both a prodigy of the imagination. Many topics, up until recently, have been considered "taboo" and left out by censorships. I do believe television does desensitize it audiences to some violence. Some ideas would have never crept its way into many minds if it had not been introduced in the comforts of someone's home. Whether people act out what they have learned is a different matter altogether. In the end, we control what we watch, and need to be held responsible for filtering out what we believe we cannot tolerate. Television is not different than any other form of outside stimuli. Television covers the mainstream society hoping to not offend its viewers. If you are ever offended or believe it may be too much for you or your family there is always an off switch.

Law #71 - Men and women have evolved into an intertwined society breaking away from the traditional norms. Women have found their places from the structured corporate world to following political ambitions; while at the same time; many men have found themselves in the domesticated households. We all are stronger, healthier, and more independent. Everyone now has more opportunities then before and less stereo types to attempt to follow.

Law #72 - The old wives' tale," the way to a man's heart is through his stomach," reveals a truth within all of us. There is an element in everyone to appreciate a home cooked meal.

Law #73 - Hoping to escape in life, looking for only the free rides offered will leave you very lonely not to mention very hungry. We all can find ourselves in very unfortunate times as we fall to our feet. It is with love and hope they may be nurtured in troubled times. We never know if those we helped yesterday may be our shelter one day from the cold. No one is safe from harsh days ahead; none of us knows what tomorrow will bring. If we ever fall victim to circumstances in or out of our control, it is wonderful to know good will is present at our fingertips. In the midst of turmoil there is always a hand to catch you, sometimes we just need to look out and reach for them, and let the kind gentleness of that hand to bring us back.

Murphy Didn't Know: A Second Look

Law #74 - If you chose not to voice an opinion when one is asked of you then you forfeit the right to demand change. The same applies if you chose not to vote your beliefs and conscience. How can one complain about governmental affairs when they are not willing to look into candidates running for office? The person elected should put their personal opinions aside and do what the majority asks of them. Those whom have been placed into office are the working arms for those whom have placed responsibilities and duties on them. We have the responsibility to ourselves and each other to vote as we see fit. If even our objectivity is in question, there are processes to remove what is unjust or unfair.

Law #75 - Whenever you decide to slow down and watch life pass you by, please do us all a favor by moving to the right side of the road. The left lane is for passing only. There are times when driving down life's open road it is best to stay in the right-hand lane with the top down and the windows rolled down granting the wind carte blanche to blow through your hair.

Law #76- In relation to the previous law, if you are the one in the right lane doing the whole wind thing, you need to keep your mouth closed or bugs might get stuck in between your teeth. While going over other safety tips, how about putting your seat belt before beginning any journey. There are reasons states have created laws requiring the use of safety belts. Few people have the intent of dying in an accident, but like most of life's trials, things can happen that we did not plan. Think for yourself, do the math, how many people owe their life to haven being restrained by a seat belt during an accident? We all lose people that have touched us and we will mourn for the loss. There is no sense in giving fate a hand up to take something or someone so important away from us. We all just need to use our heads. Speaking of using your head, protect your head by using a helmet when riding a bike. Iman accident, whom is at fault is rather meaningless when not everyone goes home that night.

Law #77 - Despite popular opinion, being rude, crude, disrespectful, or even just plain being mean to someone is not cool. If there are any questions, please go back to the beginning and start at #1, I believe you may have missed a few things.

Law #78 - You will never be able to see the goodness of others until you are able to see the goodness in yourself. Too many people are down on themselves, fighting the imperfections masked to the public. Some of these qualities that you may

Murphy Didn't Know: A Second Look

find as horrid, others may find to be what makes you the person they care for.

Law #79 - Everyone has their good days, better days and of course their bad days. Some days it is more difficult to keep your chin up through the chaos pushing you down. Find comfort in realizing the agitation does not have to dictate your serenity. The bleak circle must stop eventually, so why not close it right now. There is nothing wrong with finding peace even as waves come crashing on you. Even if this means one day of indulging in a field of happiness, it is about time you be good to yourself.

Law #80 - Looking back into history it is very easy to pick out people that have defined mankind. Often, we marvel over their determination and resolve placing these martyrs beyond Mount Olympus. Searching for any personal validation in the midst of such enormity seems inconsequential. They were never greater than any others, it is they dealt well with what they had. A leader is never better than those that follow them. Whether any one name is remembered throughout future generations, we are still all individuals filled with fears, dreams, hopes, and ambition fueling and determining the immortal conscience of tomorrow.

Kristin Blizzard

Your journey may take you to the heights of even of Mount Olympus.

Law #81 - Within the boundaries of competition always lays a desire for victory and fear of defeat. Often people are too quick to congratulate those who dominate the others or those who seem to fit naturally in the lens of the media. A champion should be measured by their performance on and off their field of play. The "great ones" are idolized from an unaware and ignorant audience. Whether others realize these immortal legends of past and present are ordinary people with ordinary lives does not take away the responsibility everyone has to make the attempt to provide a moral character when in the public eye. People that are unable to fulfill their responsibility and obligations are not worthy to remain in the spotlight. With an appeal to the purity and compassionate nature of these distinguished few, I humbly remind everyone, we need to honor the mass that placed you on the pedal stool and remember you too once looked up into the stars and dreamed.

Law #82 - In the midst of dilemma we become venerable to the scrutiny from critics. Due to lack of confidence, the fear of failure and the fear of succeeding intertwine with the fear of the unknown. Fear can be a metaphorical wall, but walls can always be climbed or knocked over.

Murphy Didn't Know: A Second Look

Maybe the answer to overcoming your fears begins and ends with believing in yourself and those that believe in you.

Law #83 - Life does have a tendency of throwing curve balls when least expected. Realistically what can you do? Sometimes you need to be ready to swing and whatever life throws at you. There is always room for a bit of luck.

Law #84 - Pulling a wedgie out of your pants is very similar to pulling a rabbit out of a hat. In both scenarios, there will be plenty of people pointing, giggling, and laughing. In either occasion in the event anything becomes stuck, things can go downhill from there. Perhaps a more private surrounding would be practical in making any necessary adjustments.

Law #85 - I do hope the concept of perseverance remains a vial burning need within. Think of the possibilities of potential and fortitude if we give fate a chance. Risking repetition, I do encourage everyone to endure the challenge and look for the strength to chase your desires and dreams.

Law #86 - One thing I cannot stress enough is our need to let go of the things we cannot control. It is a fact that as people, we will find ourselves hurt by the pains of life. We work to overcome the pain we feel, only to notice after the emotional wounds begin to heal, we trip and fall, reopening it all over again. There are those times when the past cannot help but to resurface, we all have a responsibility to ourselves to deal with the issues, to the best of our capabilities. It takes the best and worst of times to build and grow. Every day we begin a new life, those reminders from days before are from another life. Today is always the most important day of your life, yesterday cannot be changed and tomorrow is awaiting the decisions you make today.

Law #87 - When you feel life pumping from deep with inside you, when you feel the electricity pulsating and stimulating your every desire, and when you feel the fire inside burning the flame of passion, the time set out to accomplish your goals has arrived. Let the inspiration and initiative dispel problems by creating alternative solutions. The idea of life is to live.

Law #88 - As darkness surrounds you and you have no clue as to what may be right in front of you, I offer two suggestions: 1. Try to reach out to get a feel for what may lay ahead; 2. Turn on a light. Otherwise, you run the risk of running smack in the middle of a wall.

Murphy Didn't Know: A Second Look

Law #89 - In theory I would rather be poor and proud then to be rich with no purpose. Most people prefer a tender juicy filet mignon to a hamburger. I can enjoy the finer things life has to offer while I remember the cold nights of poverty. Whether this makes me a better person for it, will be determined by what I do from now on, with what I have learned.

Law #90 - If we are so "high tech," then why do we have so many remote controls? Perhaps we have stretched innovation and convenience a little too far. There is nothing wrong in developing for a better life as long as people do not lose the ability of function.

Law #91 - Using the mighty lock and key, you are doing one of two things. Either you are hoping the lock will create intimidation to a thief due to the fear of apprehension or you are appealing to the good conscience and nature of the honest. It is possible if you place such a high demand on security, you can draw attention to your fears and raise awareness to your situation. I do hope that if your good intention to be safe does backfire, you look for a means of protection more practical and less flamboyant.

Law #92 - As much as I enjoy finding humor in life, I know that not every punch line is funny. The severity of one's pain does not decline because there was no intent to injure the other person.

Law #93 - As societies have evolved, they have intertwined and borrowed from each other's culture. **The genealogy should be traced through generations if only to embrace the differences and similarities between different cultures. In the vast American "melting pot," every culture is represented within our society. We are all a part of each other. The miracle f the human spirit is: nothing can stop the goodness that flows in all of us.** Perhaps it is the prosperous attempt to remain isolated and divided from those who are different, that retains the charm of us not accepting ourselves.

Law #94 - The theory of what does not kill us only makes us stronger is: well, wrong. There is a lot of pain felt by so many people and whether or not it makes anyone stronger never really matters. Life sometimes may seem so cold and calculated to deliver us but another blow I am unable to see any benefit from having made it through the circumstance. It is the lessons that we learn by experience that defines what if anything may be beneficial. We all may live through a global disaster but if we fail to learn from the ordeal then the tragedy is doomed to repeat itself. We all will have many hours of heartache. There will be times a new light in life will shine down unto you and you will prosper from having made it through the rough times. There also maybe the times when no sense will come from what has happened. All there is for anyone to do during those times is to console each other, find support in each other, and grieve together.

Law #95 - For the most part, I do believe the public has a right to know what is going on around them. If people are not aware of their surroundings, they do not have the ability to make proper decisions in regards what they believe is best for them. However; I also do believe that people have a righto privacy. Everyone has a different story to tell. It is up to that person to decide if his or her story should be told.

Law #96 - Daring to challenge possibilities is one way to look for alternate solutions. If you are not listening, you might not be aware of the question at hand. It is good to ask when you do not know the answer, and good to answer when you do. Everyone will not always agree, but at the least, we can all agree that we have challenged ourselves, raising our minds to the next level.

Kristin Blizzard

Law #97 - Today is an excellent day to rejoice in reflection. Whether you have good fortune staring at you or not, there is always good in everyone's life. There is always a reason to be thankful for what you do have, even if itis not what you may prefer. I watch as others allow the despair, pain, and anger loom almost as if they do not see it is ok to be happy. I have yet to see happiness delivered to me in a box with the label indicating total happiness is inside. It is in everyday life, normally the smaller things that might normally go unnoticed.

Law #98 - There are two types of people that I am very uneasy with: the whiny and mentally bloated. To hear the endless complaints, the paranoia, the conspiracies existing only to taunt their everyday life infuriates me. Some people believe the rest of the world is standing in the distancing waiting for the perfect time to execute a military strike in hopes of ruining their life. I do have compassion for these people; imagine never finding peace. The other groups of people that boil my blood are those who are mentally bloated. Ignorance is never to be excused. I am referring to those whom are blessed with the capabilities but due to their ignorance, they choose to remain trapped in their dormant state of existence. If you fall into either of these two categories, I offer a few suggestions for you: 1)

Murphy Didn't Know: A Second Look

please open your eyes and grab a hold of someone's hand you trust. You need to look around; you have already missed so much. 2) When you do talk to other people, try to look into their eyes. 3) Have faith in yourself; there is never a troubled time that any one has to face it alone. There is so much out there, all you have to do is get the courage to open your eyes to see it.

Law #99 - The function of a journalist is to locate the news and to report on it. So much trust has been lost from the editorial views broadcasted one very subject. There is a responsibility from the people reporting on the current events as well as from the viewers. Unfortunately, the media is enslaved to commercial endorsement, until the ratings are no longer the first priority, viewers must search out to discover and sift out the opinions from the facts.

Law #100 - To all whom have stood up to rise to any occasion, I take my hat off to you. I respectfully bow to you whether you believe in the greatness you believe you have attained or not. Even in the worst circumstances, you did have the courage to stand up and take life on, and without doubt you have earned the right to realize in the end, you made it.

Law #101 - I hope you are presently utterly enthralled and mentally stimulated reading this book; however, you need to set it down even if it is for one minute. Life is not a book that can be opened at your leisure. AS conveniences in our lives increase with the development of technology, somethings vanish just as quickly as they appear. Go catch the sun setting as Mother Nature paints another priceless masterpiece.

Law #102 - Assuming the responsibility of raising children is the most demanding and rewarding commitment one ever makes. Raising a child is difficult at best, with many hours of agony, worry, fear, and of course, the many lessons of patience. Too often, we hear parents referring to their children as mistakes or lapses of judgment. Children are gifts that blossom into miracles. Parents and children have the opportunity to have a relationship that grows from love and respect. In the heated moments please remember that both of you always grow, typically children idolize their parents and just want to be along their side of them and prove they are worthy just like you are.

Law #103 - The time will come when there is nothing left but for you to close your eyes and trust in something you cannot see. I am not saying there is but one true religion. It is about having faith in you and having faith in something greater than yourself. We have all done our share of regretfully shameful deeds. Have faith in the fact that people are good yet we have the tendency of that dumbfounded foot entering our mouths. Trust that you makegood decisions and then by doing so, you inspire and encourage others around you to do the same.

Law #104 - After having the world within the grasp of my fingertips, I have learned the world has everything to offer. From the glamorized historical castles in Europe to the endless sands of the desert, each one possesses its own splendor. With the amazing sights I have seen, I believe this country is the best country to live in. To sit and ponder the richness of such a short history in comparison with every other nation validates what our ancestors had in thought when creating this amazing land of freedom. These simple everyday people stepped into heroic lives, as they believed in something greater themselves, they believed in us. All countries are joining this global world. We are all becoming a part of a larger melting pot. Our past is a reflection of the hopes and ideals we support today. As we witness others negating the concept that all people are created equally, we must realize

that even a fool is allowed to voice their thoughts.
You may listen and even agree if you choose, but
then again to the extremist, everyone is on a lower
level. Even in the land of the free, people are
allowed to denounce what provides them the right
to do so. I suppose in the end a fool can shed light
on the irony of a situation, even if it is them
becoming the prop that illustrates the joke.

Law #105 - Whether people are willing to admit it
or not, fake breasts are kind of like fake cheese at a
party, no one really knows exactly what is in there,
and no one wants to be the first to point it out.

Law #106 - Respect those whom have seen you
through the good and bad times. They deserve
your loyalty and you deserve theirs. They are the
people that made the commitment to stand by you.
Sometimes people do not agree. When you look at
your friends and they are on your very last nerve,
there comes a time you need to forgive and forget
it. That is what true friends do. Keep in thought as
beautiful as true friendship may be, there are
somethings that go beyond the line. You still may
forgive the act, but regaining in the friendship may
not be in your best interest. You need to do what is
best for you. Your friend that has stood by you is
your friend because you both trusted each other
enough to stand together.

Murphy Didn't Know: A Second Look

Law #107 - My family and friends have typically always supported me and stood by me in things I have done. For them I am most thankful. It is never easy for a parent to watch as their children have grown up and still face obstacles. The family structure is the most enduring relationship and bond two people can share. It does demonstrate how powerful love can be and what it can overcome. It really does not matter if you are three or a hundred and three; it is always nice to know there is someone in your corner at all times.

Law #108 - If you are guilty of plagiarizing other's opinions you are not only doing yourself an injustice, you are also crippling your potential. We all need for the sake of our own sanity to have opinions and the voice to express them. If you take the time to listen to others as you voice your thoughts, you might begin to see what you believe is not far from what everyone else believes. Too often, we shut others out or ourselves out in fear of disagreeing with others.

Law #109 - Parenting is a tough job with little in the way of thanks and praise. It is most definitely difficult for the single parent homes regardless of what you may have or know. For two parent homes, it is not a walk in the park either. I wish you good luck and patience in whatever times you find yourself.

Law #110 - From our first crushes to our high school sweet hearts; these people have allowed us to encounter a taste of relationships. Some people do wind up spending 50 years with their first love. For some, it is just the beginning of spell bounding tale filled with heartache and heartbreak. Some people may be waiting for that special love to enter their life, while others are not as willing to wait for the prince to fall off his horse. Life does not always send us in the directions we may wish for; sometimes we are thrown off our desired course. That is when we need to be reminded, we as people seem to ask for what we wish for, not what we need. In love, it may take 20 years with the wrong person before we figure out who that right person is.

Law #111 - It seems that every generation blames the one before for all that is wrong with the world. We blame them for the resources that we have been depleting, the wars we do not see fit to fight in, and the hatred installed from birth of people we have never met. This pain has become a right of passage for every next generation. As we ourselves spent our youth vowing to never repeat the same mistakes we witnessed, we pass the torch lit from decades before. Our prejudices become the fuel of

Murphy Didn't Know: A Second Look

hatred of those we treasure and offer to protect their inheritances. What worked for us two hundred years ago, may not work for us today. Laws can change as long as we continue with the spirit of freedom. If the majority sees it necessary to change existing laws to preserve equality then so be it. However; it does seem as we evolve into a modern civilization I do see an increase in the need for laws. The more we advance it appears we need more protection from predators. If we just treated others with the same respect we would like for ourselves, it would seem the world would be a better place altogether. Now we are using the rights of the people to remain ignorant as we pass laws that separate people's rights. We are incorporating laws to include hate. Freedom is a belief that all people have the right to be free; however, too often if one's life style does not stay within the norms of society, they can become a social deviant facing criminal charges. One day we will have to either get over our differences and accept people for who they are or we will face prosecution before a crime is even committed.

Law #112 - The battle of the sexes will never end. Currently, women are working just as hard as men do. The "man's job" is far from over; it has just changed a bit. Today women are as capable of providing for the family as the man stays home with the children. With technology providing commercialism more families are turning to a two income family which means both parents need to work together to provide for the children. There are single mothers and fathers doing what they must to get by. There is no guarantee a child will be the better when raised by either parent. People may question what the world is coming to: my reply is we are simply growing up.

Law #113 - There are a few things worse than catching the proverbial foot in the mouth. A simple way to avoid such a disaster is to not speak out of turn. If you would like others to listen to your thoughts, you need to listen to them. Not all "causes" are actual issues that must be dealt with. Use your head and decide for yourself. Having a different opinion then everyone else may mean you have the solution or it could mean you are finding answers for questions that no one else is asking.

Law #114 - If you decide to never line up for a race, then you are safe from the possibility of defeat but you then forego the sheer chance of winning. You may feel safe away from the field of play and in every moral aspect, you still might lose more then you could have if you actually tried. As long as you try, you do gain more then you could ever lose. The last time I checked we do have a do-over button that we make use of when we have regret later on in life.

Law #115 - Time is the most precious possession any of us will even have when we figure into how much time we actually have even given the best case scenario. Not one blissful moment should ever be emitted from memory, not one moment should ever be handed over or lost in the mayhem of daily life.
Even with the bad memories, we get to remember the goodness that we sought after: the people that touched us along the way of surviving. Often as we grow older, we look back and figure in what we might change if we had it all to do over. The truth is if any of us altered one event, significant or not, we would change the person we are today. If you can see something in yourself, you would rather change, then as long as you breathe, you have the ability to change whom you are inside.

Law #116 - Driving a car does not require status, just a little attitude. It would be quite convenient if everyone had twenty different cars to choose from that would show other drivers what mood they are in. Driving is everyday people working together in harmonious independence. If we could code our moods by what vehicle is being driven then everyone would know whether it is best to pass or to politely wait. The epidemic of road rage will continue until we gain the ability to read the minds of all of the other motorists. Until that time does occur, it is best to exercise caution and patience while on the road.

Law #117 - Tomorrow if you wake up and you feel the need to jump right back under the covers and hide from the world; then it is a great time to phone friend. I hope you never lose hope in any situation as we may often forget no situation is ever hopeless. Things may turn out to be not as scary as the first impression. I hope no one has ever lied to you by telling you how fair and easy life is. Life is lined with struggles, obstacles, and triumph as we get through the rocky times. If you can look into any situation, see all possibilities that lay ahead and the probability of them happening and still face the problem, then fear subsides and you own the situation. Friends are an awesome support system when feel like a problem is bigger than you can handle. Friends can be with you in harsh times, but they cannot conquer your fears, that task is up to you.

Law #118 - A camera is a tool to capture a piece of history forever. Every picture is a piece of the puzzle of life. It would be a shame for it not to come out after all the effort and thought you put

Murphy Didn't Know: A Second Look

forth. Some advice for those wishing to partake in the capturing of times, take the lens cap off prior to snapping the picture. For some odd reason, pictures tend to come out much better that way.

Law #119 - To give and take is so versatile. As you give a gift, you also receive the gift of acceptance from the other person as well as the gift of giving. As to who actually receiving the better of the two gifts depends on your outlook.

Law #120 - Along the lines of giving and receiving, the thought and love are put into finding the gift that suits the person that counts. How awesome is it when someone cares enough to get to know your likes and dislikes?
Those gifts remain even years after the gift was originally given.

Law #121 - There is the perfect place for everyone on this Earth. This is our home and our future. We need to take care and use wisely what we do have before we throw everything away. Once we have stripped away the natural blessings, we will have nothing to work with. Perhaps more resources are necessary to figure how to reuse our consumption rather then what we can do with what is left when we are done. People in everyday life are learning that we may be facing the greenhouse effect. This term is now heard on an everyday basis. We do know that what we are using we will run out at some point in time. There is a level of greed in every generation in knowing that our generation has not caused this nor will we see everything depleted. Others would have you look into your children's eyes, for we are creating a world very different for them. Even if our eyes do not bear witness, our blood will flow when the suffering begins.

Law #122 - Never put you above or below anyone else. No one is better or worse than others, we are all just people trying to survive. If you have committed a crime then it is up to the law to place you where justice sees fit.
It is human error to cast those away because of simple differences. That kind of intolerance was run out of town a century ago.

Law #123 - Everyone needs to confide in someone eventually. It is good to release that pent up frustration. A good friend knows the difference between built up tension and the endless ranting and raving. Voice your thoughts and shout to the moon if you see it fit, just make sure to use good judgment while doing so.

Murphy Didn't Know: A Second Look

Law #124 - The best part of bad luck is there has to be good luck thrown in the mixture for there to be any bad. A bad run cannot last forever. I am not making any promises to what your future may hold, but I am showing you there may be another way to look at any situation. Until you have the ability to know exactly what the world holds in store for tomorrow, you can always hold your head up and hope that tomorrow will be a better day.

Law #125 - Advice is one of those things that people do mean well, however; it is not always necessarily taken very well. We love our friends and family, and would like nothing more than to protect them. It does not matter how much we may want to save them from the evil deeds of the world, they need to experience life for themselves. Some people do not learn from other's mistakes and some do not even learn from their own. The best thing you can do for the both of you is to be their friend in the end. If they fall and hurt themselves, you can be there to wipe the dust off and try to help them find the courage to try again. Whether you know with absolute certainty what is about to happen, they may need to feel the effects from falling. It is harder to watch someone you love gets hurt then for it to happen to yourself. Hopefully, nothing but their ego will be bruised. All one can do is give people the options with whatever is going on, but how they respond is up to them. They need to make the decisions based on where they are in life.

Law #126 - There are times you might be listening to the radio, you hear a song, and it feels as if the artist is dedicating just to you. That is ok. Who is to say if it was written for you or not? Other than the writer, I doubt if anyone knows for certain. If a song enchants a particular mood to come out in you, if it feels good, then where is the harm in allowing them to sing to you until your heart is content?

Law #127 - We all know every day we have the ability of learning something new. There are so many little lessons life teaches us, and even some big ones too. There is never enough time for one person to have learned everything. Imagine living in the times when fire was feared from lack of knowledge. In the future, we may laugh as we recall our present sophistication. Once we have figured our present four walls, then it is time to move on to the next set of four walls.

Law #128 - If you become so afraid of death, you begin to stop living, then chances are you have already died in spirit. There is a time each of us must face up to mortality's grasp. We all need to look at what we have done with what we have been given. The quality of life can exceed in importance over the quantity. I would much rather have the conscience of a great person for one day then to live a hundred lives without purpose.

Law #129 - As you wonder into the unexplored, you may come across and unbeaten path. Chances are you are not the first to have actually seen it, and it has been preserved as a gift passed to you and for you to pass on to others. A day may come when you have a need for that very path. Once it has destroyed then it will only remain in memories. Preservation is one of those things we hear our parents talking about, typically followed by the phrase, "If I only knew."

Law #130 - Once you are able to feel the difference between sympathy and empathy you will begin to see differences in yourself. You may have sympathy for someone in trouble, and even desire nothing more than to help those in need. Having sympathy shows how good of a person you are. Having empathy is actually feeling the pain others are going through. Their pains become yours. You will not be able to help those if you yourself are too far into the wound. There is enough for you to bear without adding other's pains.

Law #131 - You cannot help others if you are unable to help yourself first. If you are taking on too much, you may be increasing the risks to yourself and in the end, you will no longer be capable of helping others nor yourself. We all need to strengthen ourselves before taking on the problems of the world. As good as your intentions might be, you may wind up doing more harm than good.

Law #132 - Losing someone hurts us all; it is in that pain that we must hold onto one another. One loss is always one too many. It is senseless to push away the other people in your life; they should be there for you when you need them the most.

Law #133 - We gain wisdom two ways: experience and knowledge. Times may require you to use both and still may not provide you with the wisdom to get through the situation. If you ever find yourself unsure throughout your journey, then like when we are lost, you may need to stop and ask for directions. Chances are you and the person you find to ask to come from slightly different paths even though the finish line may be the same. It may be the difference of a single second, but that one second may be what changes the impression you leave.

Murphy Didn't Know: A Second Look

Law #134 - Take note to all of your surroundings all of the time. It is not for your safety alone, but for all those that around you. We need to look out for one another in case the worst of circumstances does circumvent. Not only will you know what exactly has happened but you also may be the one that sees the reason why.

Law #135 - Providing a safety net from life's threat may mean sometimes you need to leave out your personal opinion. There is always a level of personal security necessary to reassure that the independence of the individual is free to follow its own course. If the time does arrive that you feel threatened and need to find shelter, your instinctive warning system will alarm to let you know there is a problem. At the time your fears have raised concerns, you need to evaluate the circumstance and act with thought as you deliver yourself from whatever the situation is at hand.

Law #136 - Hopefully, most people find the piercing sound of a 44magnum very startling. The real trick is forgetting the sound as it haunts you for years to come. In a fraction of a second, lives are altered as the cold raw force rips through the air. That ripping sound can taunt memories and leaving victims scarred for life. This is just like every other severely traumatic event and seeking professional help is the first step in getting past it.

Law #137 - Irony brings out the familiarity in extremities, yet the humorous side is in the possibility of an event reoccurring as the event has been resolved. A common belief is life is filled with random coincidences rather than a designed fate. Perhaps a day will come when we will have a better understanding of exactly why things happen; on the other side of the coin, maybe it is not our place to know.

Law #138 - After living with a person for an extended period of time, the two of you may begin to pick up each other's habits, expressions, and even behaviors. I hope that you are picking up the little things that made you want to be around them in the first place. It is easy to find flaws or differences in how you may react. Just remember you once did find them worthy enough to enter the relationship in the first place.

Law #139 - An artist is destined to live the life demanded by their art. Perhaps it is not fate; perhaps the subconscious mind flirts in attempt to expand itself. The pains of life are often painted on a canvas or whispered through a sonnet. To create a masterpiece, you must first look to what inspires you. There are often times when tragedy reins in and creates an emotional melancholy easily represented. I believe people live their lives in defiance, creating the lines of where they wish to go or how they wish for into be portrayed.

Law #140 - It is not possible to proficiently defend an idea when it does not support your own. Even the best prepared cannot always contend with the passion the other side might have. If you find yourself in the middle of a situation you do not know about, then it is best left for the parties involved. If there is someone that would like your help, he or she will ask for it. It is awesome that you are primed to help at a moment's notice; however, it is best before doing so, make sure it is wanted.

Law #141 - Having and using common sense has apparently become somewhat of a rarity. This may be one of the biggest reasons people have their feelings hurt so often. I think we should all try to play nicely with others, but even I admit; there are some people out there that make it rather difficult. Everyone should be given some room for error. When your patience is low and you feel the steam building, take a minute to relax, we are all people, and people make mistakes.

Kristin Blizzard

Law #142 - There once was a time when you could give your word and that was enough for people. Now people need to protect themselves, it seems like where ever we turn, there is someone out there that tries to "get one over." It is a sad day when we compromise ourselves and lose sight of our own words and beliefs.

Law #143 - There is absolutely nothing in the world that says everyone needs to wake at the crack of dawn. I trust all the "day people" will be able to handle what needs to be done in the morning, and they may also rest well knowing that when the moon is lighting the sky that I will be there rooting the stars to fill the heavens. Once upon a time, there was life only after 6am and before 9pm. We welcome the next millennium with our lives together on global platform. We are more efficient and have the energy when we operate within the time that best suits our bodies.

Law #144 - Parents do ask some odd questions. It seems like once a child is brought into the world, common sense becomes void. Having questions and concerns is common; I would be more concerned if there were no questions. No one is perfect so why would you believe there would be no mistakes in raising a child?

Murphy Didn't Know: A Second Look

Law #145 - People that have committed crimes against society are known as criminals. There are people that lobby for those incarcerated asking for more rights within the prison walls. Should people that have committed crimes against society be entitled to a better life then their victims? At present time, prison provides cable TV, weight rooms, libraries, three meals a day, a warm bed to sleep in ECT... Poverty typically does not provide as much as our prison systems do, so how can we be surprised to find an increase in crimes? As we continue to lobby for more right for inmates, we must realize we are replacing the bars on the prisons for bars on the victims' windows. We feed the criminal's desire by not rewarding those whom choose to live respectfully. Our society inadvertently mocks those struggling to make ends meet with an honest living. Rehabilitating criminal behavior begins with a prison system that punishes intolerable behavior. We need to follow a path of fairness the wrong people, we are reinforcing someone to repeat their offence. Inmates have rights to an extent; however, if they have committed crime they should have to serve the society they violated. Overcrowding of prisons and jails are becoming all too common, perhaps if we removed the TV, basketball courts, and the weight rooms we would save in the space, save taxes payer money for the purchase and up keep of them, as well as it may discourage people to commit the crimes. The money saved could then be used to assist people in need rather then turning them to crime. We need to address why crimes are committed and put resources there rather than providing a country club lifestyle for those whom seek to injure others. Once they have made retribution for their crimes, then they should be given a second chance. How can there be justice if a criminal has a better life than those they commit the crimes against?

Law #146 - There are two sides to every story. Listen to the other side and judge it according to how it affects you, not others. If you are asked for your opinion, then before entering a verdict, view all of the facts and possibilities. When weighing in all of the evidence you need to be honest and fair to the situation. In life, there are some things black and white, yet, typically when dealing with people there is always gray in the middle. Just remember not everything happens just as it appears, there are often variables that must be calculated in the process.

Law #147 - Never let someone you love walk away. Once you have parted, you cut off the ties that once bounded the relationship. It is easy to let a quick temper ruin a beautiful thing. I would hate if pride were the reason for someone to live alone pondering, "If I only would have…"

Law #148 - If one chooses to live the life of a king: he ought to be a king. High society equals high demands. No one is going to provide you with the high life simply at your request. Everything must be paid in full. Even a mighty king must give up something before he sees the riches of his land.

Law #149 - If you have to ask yourself whether or not you should do something, then you know the answer from the get go. From the time of adulthood, people expect you to have a basic understanding of right and wrong. You are accountable for your actions. Once you decide to cross the lines in front of you, you are on your own.

Law #150 - The only kind of overnight success that exists is the kind that takes years of dedication and luck. Your goals have the possibilities of becoming reality once you realize the time necessary to achieving it. Follow the path and see where fate takes you. Things may not happen the way you prefer, but since when has any one had the ability to control their overall fate?

Kristin Blizzard

Law #151 - Technology can be our best friend or our toughest foe. There is no reason to depend on it solely to exist. We need to depend on our abilities to function and use it to increase our standard of living. We should stick to its purpose rather than seeking out opportunities to exploit it. Mankind has a history of taking things that are intended to benefit society and find a darker purpose then exploit it even further. A day will come when technology may not work, then we will need to rely on our natural instincts. Society has survived long before the many comforts of home, and it can again if needed.

Law #152 - Often people make an attempt to change public opinion for their own personal gain. We get used to these hidden agendas and then unexpectedly, someone comes along that step forward for the benefit of everyone. Listen to yourself and be open to reason. If one person can be wrong, then it is very possible 10 million people can be wrong about the something. People are swayed by those who lobby for change. If people are not receiving all of the facts, then they are not actually deciding anything. It is everyone's responsibility to search out all of the facts to both sides before determining what the right thing is.

Law #153 - I am sure that you have at least once been told to not say anything if you do not have

Murphy Didn't Know: A Second Look

anything nice to say. After hearing it from others, it should not surprise anyone, hearing again. There is enough negativity already out there.

Law #154 - Let us suppose you are following a path in life and there right front of you lies a-bomb, oh my, what should you do? You have basically three choices to choose from but only one chance to do the right one. The first choice is the proactive approach; you can attempt to disarm the bomb. While the odds of your bomb disarming training not being completed as of yet may be rather high, you might get lucky with the wires. Without doubt this would be the most explosive and adventurous but probably not the smartest approach. The second choice is the passive approach, do nothing. There is a chance the bomb might not go off, or perhaps it may miss you. The third is the reactive approach, turn and run as fast as the wind allows. To some this may be the coward's way, but if the coward survives, they do get to try again another day. If you are deciding which of these three approaches best fits you present situation then perhaps this is an excellent opportunity to see the value of having options. You may not have the know how to handle it and may need help. Sometimes there is no other choice to flea for safety sakes. You can only do what is right for you to do.

Know there is a consequence for everything you do good or bad.

Law #155 - Peer- pressure is a reality faced in every society; however, you do have the right to say no. If you do not want to follow the crowd, then you have a responsibility to yourself to say no. You have the right to be your own person and believe what you like. You may become the new trend by creating a new path for others to follow.

Law # 156 - It is feasible that even our most treasured possession are nothing but junk to everyone else. I would hate to think a prize held in so much regard could lay in the trash a month later. One man's junk is another man's treasure. We keep things for not only how they make us feel as well as what they represent. This is how price is valued. That glorious trophy now sits on the mantle collecting dust. To you this trophy may symbolize your greatest achievement while others may see it as an eye sore.

Law #157 - Everyone is allowed to have a bad day here and there. Sometimes people do not feel well, or maybe need a new pillow to end the crick in the neck. Do not let what ails you ruin your entire day. You may not behaving as bad as a day as you may think. Maybe it is a rough start to the best day of your life. Some things will never get better and the

Murphy Didn't Know: A Second Look

only thing left is to better yourself as best you can. The next thing you might know is your day gets better. All you had to do to get there was change your perception of the current situation in its entirety.

Law #158 - For every friend you might find, there may be a thousand heartbreaks around the corner. A true friend will be there to help you get past whatever the rest of the world can throw at you. Chances are, you are a friend to someone, and you make every broken promise from everyone else worth it. You just being you and standing by your friends illustrate the reasons we all need each other.

Law #159 - A diet will never hold over the long term. There are so many to choose from, we can deprive some foods to increase the body's metabolism or limit the intake of daily consumption. Weight loss has become a huge concern. Some people exercise and have great results; others try the latest fad diet. Perhaps prior to changing your life style, you should consult your family doctor. Your doctor is the best person to analyze your medical history and come up with what is healthy; after all, losing weight and being fit should be done for good health as the primary reason.

Law #160 - It is a reflection of what kind of a person you are by your willingness to battle the many injustices of the world, but there are too many for one to battle alone. Fighting everyday of your life with so much passion is a very hard life to live. Everyone owns the responsibility to better what he or she can be. If you wear yourself out early then you in your prime will have a short life.

Law #161 - There are so many people out there, some are going to be nice to you while others are going to be as harsh as they feel everyone else is to them. Before you allow yourself to fall victim to their negativity please consider where they are in relationship to you. Whatever someone says about you, it is the good inside of you that matters. There are people that will use you, hurt you, and tear you down but you do not live for them. Those are the few that spoil it for the rest of us. Just keep in mind you are not the only person that would like to see world peace, and end to hunger, and of course an end to mixed plaid.

Law #162 - There is a difference between growing up and growing old. Time moves on whether you want it to or not. Even if you fight tooth and nail, maturity will surface sooner or later. It all boils down to understanding that we will all eventually learn our lessons; therefore, we all grow up some

Murphy Didn't Know: A Second Look

time. You need to keep in mind growing older is a mental enigma. Age is rather minuscule when used to figure maturity. There are many ignorant adults functioning in society. Hopefully they are not the ones we elect to run the country.

Law #163 - Ending a relationship can be one of the hardest things you ever do. It is with much regret that our paths must part ways, but there is comfort in the good times we shared. You can never go back to the person you once were, with every relationship comes a new experience. Perhaps it is easier to say goodbye knowing hopefully you will be a better person from having the opportunity to know them. You might not have benefited the way you prefer, but never the less they have altered your course.

Law #164 - Threat of change is overcome once you have realized change was in order. People in general do not like change. There is confidence gained over repetition, as a change begins we all see our raw untried skills that we are no longer the masters of as before. Just as the primitive men before us, we slide backwards using the trial and error until atlas a breakthrough occurs. It is true the first attempt is never our best. If we feel passionate in our efforts then our many attempt of perfection is well worth the time and effort.

Law #165 - Gambling for many is an addiction, a sport, or even a sin. If you wager more than you can lose then you enter into a risk of losing your foundations. Some people are not comfortable in playing it safely and to the many loss is too high of a risk. Remember there is no such thing as a "sure thing" after all if there were it would not be a gamble.

Law #166 - Parents are the first of many role models and the impression left is what creates the mold that children will learn from. Kids will learn both good and bad habits from their parents. If you speak with a foul tongue then your child will as well. If you child watches you steal, they too will become a thief. Tomorrow belongs to the youth of today, so how can we help but nourish their minds and bodies.

Law #167 - It does not matter how hard someone tries to alter their appearance. It is what we are made of inside that should be of concern. A Pretty face is just that, but a beautiful person is everything to so many.

Law #168 - There are times when pampering yourself goes a long way. How long has it been

Murphy Didn't Know: A Second Look

since you have treated yourself to a little R & R? Perhaps you fancy a stay in a nice hotel to lounge by the pool, or perhaps sneaking off to a movie, or maybe even just taking yourself out for a nice meal. Not everyone has the funds available to splurge, so sometimes we have to work at having some fun without spending any money. A vacation may be taking a half hour lunch or maybe just stopping to smell the flowers. Self-indulgence may just be what the doctor ordered. A good attitude may be the difference between your sanity and the crazed indifference of everyday life.

Law #169 - Life is unquestionably a quest to experience. However, breaking your neck to prove or disprove a theory is not going to be the most intelligent decision on your agenda. We all need to be proactive and try our best in what we are meant to do. Not everyone is suited to be a dare devil nor is everyone suited to be a doctor. There is no shame in you living the life that is meant for you to live. I wish everyone would see how exhilarating and breathe taking life can be.

Law #170 - Everyone needs at some point to feel the love from others. Even tougher to admit is the love we have for others. Most of us would admit there are some people that have touched us and we

would go to any length to be there for them. Our very last dollar would be of no consequence if it were the dollar they needed. We pour out anything needed to improve the life of the people we know and even the faces we may never look into. It is ironic once these faces have a defined loyalty we discredit them as individuals. They become blemishes in our society and thus they no longer are privileged in our eyes. I once heard a story about a vain society whom believed they were superior to everyone that had any difference. Friends turned their back on one another and complete chaos over took them in a civilized time. Camaraderie ceased to exist. The next empire that reigned for another 100 years until they too awaited the same fate as those they oppressed before replacing them. It is all a cycle, as people are controlled by greed and jealousy, the cycle will always have the next beginning and end for some. Hopefully, our global business empire will provide enough hope and peace to insure the destruction does not continue in our day and age.
Perhaps we will be the ones that stand together regardless of language, race, or beliefs.

Law #171 - Materialism reflects the level of importance we place on replaceable items. There is nothing wrong with having quality possessions around you; it is only a concern when they become more valuable to you then everything else. Price is

Murphy Didn't Know: A Second Look

not always a determining factor when searching for quality; but it is true you do get what you pay for. I have been slightly spoiled as I indulged into the finer things in life. My parents like most just wanted the best for me and they provided what they saw was necessary and available at the time. By allowing me to bite into the best, I found a taste for quality, but also saw the need to have the best; I would have to work very hard to enjoy it. Nothing is ever out of our reach as long as we can focus on what it actually is and can grasp that it will never be handed to us, it is something we must work for.

Law #172 - If you think you are unable to handle an answer then you have no business asking the question. It is tough to hear criticism. If you are not up to an honest answer then think twice before asking for it. You may hear what you want to, you may not. There is no benefit for either person if there is no honesty. If others ask for your thoughts hopefully, you can honor them by being honest yet with diligence.

Law #173 - No matter how much you love someone, you never can control their love. People cannot control who they fall in love with. It is crazy for anyone to believe they can place a leash on love and take it out at will. At times, we may be

scratching our heads trying to figure out what went wrong. It is possible to be swept up in the moment.
That moment may last for twenty years. If separation becomes viable, then look for comfort in knowing the right relationship may lie ahead. As strong as you feel towards another person, you cannot dictate how he or she feels to the degree you desire. It does nothing positive to attempt to relive past relationships while you forego possibilities. We often hear parents stay with their spouses "for the kids." Children are not as ignorant as we may wish for them to be. Children should remain out of the equation when deciding what is best for you. A family unit may change, as does everything else in the rest of the world.
Ending a marriage has nothing to do with finding blame or punishing a culprit. Children have fears when they do not understand, but they too are people with good and bad intentions. A fantastic surprise may be awaiting all parties after the dust settles. Parents may remarry and then who knows, maybe there will be a new family or even a wonderful new friend in the end. The fact of life is we do not know what the world has yet to offer and there is no one out there with all of the answers. People do make mistakes and we are apt to fall to error. I am not saying that a divorce is the answer to anyone's problem. Sometimes it does happen that two people lose the connection and spark they once felt. In the heat of an argument, we

say things that are hurtful. Sometimes our actions speak louder than words we shout out. We never know if the person we are with is meant to be our best friend or is our soul mate.

Law # 174 - There are some things that not everyone is going to agree on. If it has nothing to do with you then why would you waste your energy and time on something that is not your concern? Who says it is the others that have the problem, in the end you might be the one missing out. None of us have the power to change other people. We can present other options and they may change their opinion.

Law #175 - A discussion is one of the best tools we have to solve problems and answer questions. If you feel you are not reaching the desired results and you choose to use force, you may lose by default. The most powerful and difficult thing to change is someone else's mind. If you present all the facts and still face the disagreement from the opposition then it maybe you or them that must rethink their positions. They may fail to see your points and vice versa due to ignorance and personal opinion. You cannot change whether someone else is ignorant to the facts, you can only realize they are not better or worse than you are because they do not see your point of view.

Law #176 - Dreaming as to what your future may hold expands the limits of possibilities one possesses. Through the turmoil, we come across moments of genius. Seize the day! If you stop wading over the smaller things and go for the glory, you might see all the dreams of you past and present coming true. If the times of brilliant ingenuity are motivated by your subconscious, then you are constructing from the daydreaming and creating realities. We spend too much time on figuring doubt into what may come that we lose the drive to push forth. Perhaps all the time spent on dreaming as a child is starting to pay off. Expand yourself by using the ideas to create paths to follow. The greatest sin you can ever commit against yourself to abandon your potential due to your fears of dreaming and succeeding, and just windup with regret for never trying.

Law #177 - The best offence is typically the best defense. It is also true if you spend all of your time defending yourself, then you may miss the chance to look at what is around you. No one should ever feel pressured to maintain a defensive wall all of the time, it is not healthy. If you have you guard up all of the time, how will you blossom into the person you should be? The times may warrant

caution, but there is also a time when we all have to
throw our hands in the air and succumb to the will
of the wind.

Law #178 - If you are standing in the way of
progress, then you must be prepared to be pushed
aside. People want to live better than they did the
day before.

Law #179 - Good will shall persevere over
negativity as long as we find goodness in everyday
life. As we watch as others debilitate those less
fortunate, it is our duty as people that share this
planet to stand up to protect the innocent. We need
to stop allowing children to believe violence is the
answer for all problems. There is not a difference
between a child shooting a child or an adult
shooting an adult, both of these scenarios have a
treacherous fate to our future. We all must have
boundaries in all levels of communication for there
to be the prosperity for peace. The vision we leave
for future generations should be illustrated with
possibility for amity. If we do not want guns in the
hands of our children then we must first set the
example for them to follow. There is a time when
we must wage a war, but this is not a battle suited
for our children to fight.

Law #180 - You can be number one at anything as long as you are willing to set the standard and adhere to the demands of maintaining that position. The pressure is always greater for those to repeat a title rather than to set out in search of the top. You can count on as long as you hold the title there will always be others out there waiting in the shadows for their chance to take the title and become champions. Once you have succeeded in taking the top of the hill, you need to prepare yourself and work even harder to remain there. Perhaps in the planning of how you will attempt to get to the top, you may also want to figure some ways to keep you at the top of your game.

Law # 181 - If you decide to stand up for a cause I hope you understand why a concern has been raised. Most people can be swayed one way or the other as long as the facts have been suppressed. If you are going to get involved, then you need to do your own research and make up your own mind from there. No one has the ability to solve a problem if we do not take the time to understand what if anything is the problem. Your best efforts can be negated if your emotions are persuaded into overlooking what your mind would normally say.

Law #182 - It is easy to place blame on those people we have a more intimate knowledge of. After people get close to us and see us for our

Murphy Didn't Know: A Second Look

weaknesses and strengths, their loyalty always becomes a question whenever a disagreement occurs. Maybe a solution is to trust in yourself more. It was your judgment that allowed that person to get close to you when you originally decided on bestowing that friendship. There was a reason in the beginning just as there may still be a reason to try to salvage your relationship now.

Law #183 - You cannot judge everyone in your future by your past. People are always going to be different. Some people are meant to be in your life and for all you know, you are meant to go off and tackle the world together. Before you can overcome any fears, you have of other people, you need to let go of the past. There is nothing wrong with keeping your guard up until you feel safe. If you give people a chance, you may be very pleasantly surprised at what you might find. Even if you hope everyone you are going to meet is bad; the truth is most will not be. Possibly, you can expand your own horizons by not categorizing the world into groups; people are far too random to set aside in groups.

Law #184 - There comes a point in time in everyone's life when we have to find the acceptance and get past what happened in the earlier days. Maybe times were tough and life was not fair; but we all know life is not always fair to begin with. Everyone has been a victim in some regards. We do not need to be a victim forever. As you raise your children, you hope you nourish them with everything they need to one day grow into good, honest, and most importantly happy adults. As children, we lead them into a world of sharing and caring for all others. As they grow up a few years down the road, we show them what it is to be humble and graceful. We expect them to understand what it is to have good sportsmanship. Then as even a few years pass, we begin to monitor them less and less until we slide on how nice they should be to others. As long as they are not breaking any rules, they are still apparently on course. Then one day we wonder if the children we hear about in the news are anything like our own. Sometimes we may have crossed lines or had others cross our lines. What was done to us or by us remains in tepas! Everyone has been hurt by someone, just as we have hurt others in the jungle known as youth. As we have grown, we have become different people.

Children today face many of the same aspects other children shared the playground from years before; but, now we are wiser and hopefully can see the faults and try to not repeat them. To the many people just like me I offer hope and some inspiration. We now have the opportunity to better and change ourselves into what we want to be. We are now good to others with the hopes that our goodness is carried on.

Law #185 - Every civilization has in it very different customs. Some may seem rather odd to you, but you still need to respect others as they life as they see fit. After living in the Midwest for many years, I still have not found the glory in cow tipping. Apparently, individuals gather into group to find non-suspecting animals asleep, and they "push" them over. Amazing how some people may mock others for stomping on grapes barefoot and see nothing wrong with pushing an unsuspecting animal over to only run away for dear sweet life from this crazed beast. I am not saying what they do is any more or less odd then what others do, I am simply pointing out; others may view this adventure as slightly off the normal beaten path.

Law #186 - All problems have solutions. Finding the objectivity during a crisis, to prevent furthering the issue, may be the "tip of the solution." A cool head may be needed as times are heated. With the many issues we face today, I believe we should all work together to solve some of them. Without the insight, you might not only cripple those whom may have been the best at finding solutions, but we may further the damage and increase the recovery time. Until we unlock every mystery in the universe, there will remain several options: nothing is written in stone per say.

Law #187 - For one reason or another there lays in all of us a desire to have what we cannot have. Often we lose interest in what we have in the attempt to study what everyone else has. The power of jealously is an aggressive force that debilitates those in search of self-esteem. Everyone has different physical and emotional belongings other may look at with envy. Itis good to have goals in order to gain something. However, a physical possession never defines who you as a person.

Law #188 - An army is only as great as its leaders. A leader is as strong as it's weakest soldier. If we lead the chain of command into the ground then there is where our destiny lies. To improve yourself, you will need to learn to bring others up to your level. Sometimes we are forced to work with people that care less about the job at hand for the greater good. A soldier's job is to follow the order from his or her commander. A basic fundamental in life is we all must survive. This often means ending the fun and doing a job to the best of our abilities no matter of our greeting or liking the task at hand.

Murphy Didn't Know: A Second Look

Law #189 - There is nothing wrong with an active approach when working towards the future. The future is coming whether or not you are ready for it. We all should look at the possibilities in store. Everyone does have a future no matter how long or short it may be, and we all must see the glory that goes with whatever time we have left.

Law #190 - Once in a while, we need to relax and take some time for ourselves. As an adult, we may choose to unwind with a drink or two. Also as adults, we have responsibility to insure if we decide to do this, we follow basic rules. If you drink in excess, then you should not drive. Many bars will be more than happy to call you a cab; some will even happily pay for your ride home. There is no such thing as a good reason to drive after drinking. Another good piece of advice is if you are going out to a local club, it is safer to go with someone else. Unfortunately, there are predators waiting for the right victim to drop something in an unsuspecting drink. Another piece of advice is to limit what you tell people about yourself. Avoid giving personal details like your phones number, address, and home telephone number. I hope everyone can have a good time and relax when you can, just please do so while using your head.

Law #191 - As you find yourself enjoying a wonderful meal at a local restaurant, you may take notice to the excellent quality of the food and how it rivals the best home cooked meal. Then it does not take long to notice the dishes are also not your problem for the evening. It is a nice change to let others slave over the inferno for once. The only thing left to do is kick your feet up and enjoy every minute of it.

Law #192 - If one is to compare building trust to building a bridge, one would find many similarities. The foundations of both take time and hard work to start from the ground up. The many secrets friends share between each other would be the fasteners. The sleepovers filled with endless gossip would be the support beams. We give a little of ourselves as we talk, then with more trust comes extending the bridge until it stretches across the river. Sometimes a storm may threaten or even knock a bridge out. After the damage is done, the bridge like the trust, must be cleaned out and slowly rebuild. This is the long run will make both the bridge and the friendship stronger. Just keep in mind both can be fixed as long as both of you are willing to invest the time and hard work.

Law #193 - A true shopper lives for the thrill of the hunt. A bargain shopper just remembers to bring

Murphy Didn't Know: A Second Look

the coupons. Imagine what would happen if the true shopper met up with the bargain shopper.

Law #194 - If you believe you will never use more than 7% of your brain then your brain is only that 7%. Instead of accepting that as fact, why not try for more? You need to find resources inside of yourself to unlock more.
Science is a tool we use to figure out the answers to questions. If we allow it to define us, then logic becomes the enemy.

Law #195 - If you would like your children to learn, it begins with the example you show them. We have movies and TV that replaces the basics.
If adults are not willing to spend the time to open a book, then how is a child supposed to learn reading fundamentals?

Law #196 - In our democratic government we have a checks and balanced system. This is the same concept found in most successful businesses, nations, and even marriages. It is different bodies that check and recheck each other to insure a sense of fairness. Not every mistake is an intentional mishap; there have been reports of people making honest mistakes.

Law #197 - If you love someone then part of loving them is loving them for who they are. If you decide to dedicate your life to another person, then you are agreeing any differences you may have with them, they are acceptable. No one has the right to change their other half after committing themselves to one another. It is unfair to demand change after you have already made the commitment. If you cannot live with the person, you are with and they are unwilling to change or modify to adapt to your concerns, then you are the one that needs to keep looking.

Law #198 - In the heat of an argument we often say things we would never say otherwise. You can never take back the pain you caused; all you can do is hope they forgive what has been said. Instead of relying on the other's goodwill, perhaps a better idea is to step back and look at the situation. It is good to give second or third chances; but there comes a point in time when you need to forgive and just let go. If it is meant to be then there is no force strong enough to keep you apart. You may give 100 second chances if the problem is manageable. If you are unable to cope with the issue, then it might be time for you to just move on.

Law #199 - There is comfort in a known, safe, and unchanged environment. As comfortable as it may be, if you need a little excitement then rock the

Murphy Didn't Know: A Second Look

boat. You need to be ready for whatever comes your way. Everyone needs to stir things up once in a while, after all, we do all need some change to break up our daily routines.

Law #200 - During the course of our lives, we will all encounter pain; therefore, there is never a need to inflict suffering on innocent people. I can assure you there are far more interesting and productive things you could be spending your time on.

Law #201 - With the many people you share this planet with; you can count on there being plenty of people waiting with opposition. You have the right to pursue happiness, as does everyone else. Few people prefer war and hunger to a utopian society. The chance at happiness begins with you ignoring what everyone desires and look at yourself and find exactly what it is that makes you happy and go from there.

Law #202 - During the merry times of the holiday season, it appears people get to be a bit pushy. You need to be careful to not run into any of Santa's little helpers. You never know when the pressure gets to be more than they can handle and then the elves go postal!

Kristin Blizzard

Law #203 - What comes around, goes around. If you think before speaking and think before acting, you will avoid a lot of embarrassment. If you plan everything you may feel like you are losing the edge, but it is always better to lose the edge then to lose the game.

Law #204 - Normality in society is simply a phrase; normal is the setting on a washing machine. If you have to fit in the "norm," then you like everyone else needs to find his or her individualism.

Law #205 - I have noticed many similarities in the majority of different religions. One may see the likeness from Buddhism to Christianity, and even to Zoroastrianism: noting the basic belief in a presence battling over an evil spirit. Every religion follows its own beliefs and customs as they pray using a different name; but who really knows if He may be one God that answers to many names?

Law #206 - If you live your life for everyone else, you might see such sorrows as you begin to realize that time never turns back. We all need to see the gifts that we are given today and cherish them as if time exists only to hold such treasured possessions so dear. Time is a continuous line that will always reach further then our arms.

Murphy Didn't Know: A Second Look

Law #207 - I do like believing people to be of a kind heart and use common sense. Talk about being disappointed occasionally. I was living in Colorado at the time: as I walked into the kitchen, I noticed the stove on med-high with a pot of water warming. I did ask why the water was not on high. For some reason, they were concerned if it were turned up, then maybe the temperature would be too hot for the water.

Law #208 - Personal reflection can be a great tool in coping with issues. Journaling you daily thoughts and concerns is a way to review your everyday progress, as well as provides excellent reading material if ever in the nostalgic mood.

Law #209 - After sharing an extended time with others as friends, the hardest thing is to realize sometimes people change and friends need to go their separate ways. As difficult as it is to let a friend go, there is a time when self-preservation must become the priority. Perhaps people grow out of certain behaviors and refocus their energy. For whatever reason you deem it necessary, if it is your best interest, then you may have to do the unthinkable and walk away.

Law #210 - Everyone enjoys one form of excitement or another. However, some push excitement further. Having the need to feel threatened in order to achieve the thrill is when it becomes a dangerous addiction that needs to be treated. Most people would never think about jumping from an airplane without a parachute. Of course in that example most people on the planet would never seriously even consider it. Even in extreme sports there are some risks and safety concerns that are always a factor. I enjoy rock-climbing but I would never go without the ropes.

Law #211 - There is never a magical age when parents' separating does not affect the children. There are many emotions that need to be dealt with. It is normal for children of any age to feel torn as they watch as their parents end their relationship. Blame, fear, misplaced loyalty, over compensation; confusion, anger, and even depression are just a small list of issues children may deal with. For some, watching a daily battle between their parents may be harder to get through then a divorce. Parents do not have the luxury of whether or not they wish to be respectful of the other. Children see and hear everything, and without proper discussion, they will fill in the blanks parents leave out. People get married very early, normally before they have an idea of who they are as individuals. With parents working

Murphy Didn't Know: A Second Look

together, there is no reason for children to be unable to find peace with the situation. Simple reminders and reassurances go a very long way in realizing the family unit may alter but the parents still love as parents always have.

Law #212 - A true fan will love their team in good times and in bad times. It would be nice if people would extend that loyalty to other people. Unconditional love reigns above all else. We should feel free to be the person we are without fear of how the world will look at us. I am willing to let others see me for what I am and what my beliefs are. Not everyone is going to agree with everything, but in reality, it is not his or her place to either agree or disagree.

Law #213 - Some secrets are meant to be held in the highest of confidence and some are meant to be shared. They should be thought of with the highest regard when someone else thinks enough of you to entrust a piece of them that they do not feel comfortable sharing with the rest of the world. Something so tender that has been shared through the bonds of trust and friendship, is a gift. I have trusted my friends with a lot, but I know what I have shared with them is kept in secret because of the kind of person they are. I cherish my friends now as I did when I wanted them to know me for who I was. I have been very lucky to have many wonderful people in my life, and I am glad now as I was then when I shared part of my life with them. Even the ones that we parted ways; there is solace in the times we did spend together. If those from your past were ever truly genuine, then perhaps without publicly admitting it, they might concede that they too found comfort in the bond once shared.

Law #214 - Public education has fallen in recent years and as it continues to fall, points to the concerns we will have in the future. We have teachers that work hard for very low wages. We have new schools that would appease king yet lack the funds to upgrade older schools. All children should be provided with every possible means we have to educate them. School is the place to build academic knowledge, social skills, and even to improve the abilities to learn. The primary focus is becoming reading a book and the knowledge will absorb from there. As stimulating as it is for some to read, there is much more to a successful classroom. The day to learn is today. We need to take back the control in the classrooms and remove the disturbances not the children. There should never be tolerance of behaviors that interfere with someone learning. A child that wants to advance their education should be encouraged once they have the basics. It is very typical for parents to want a better life for their children, yet, we are not giving them the tools to do so.

Law #215 - In my world, some animals do not make the best pets. Personally, I will never have a reptile, insect, or rodent. If you require a cage to keep your pet in that may be clue #1 there may be a problem. Clue #2if people refuse to visit you at your home; it may be time to rethink what is acceptable for you to have a pet. Pets should be given love, food and shelter. All joking aside, if you have the ability to provide a good home to a pet then it is wonderful doing so.

Law #216 - Bottled water should have a toy surprise or something in it if people are going to pay $2 a bottle.

Law #217 - One of the best things about becoming an adult and having your own space is your ability to do what you want to. If you decide to open a cereal box to only take the toy out or have ice cream for breakfast that is your decision to make. As you get older, your body may decide for you what you can or cannot eat. You may see a reward after you eat certain foods or your body may punish you after eating other foods.

Kristin Blizzard

Law #218 - A strong offence does provide an edge over your adversary. Theoretically, a strong offence may put others on a mental alert status keeping them from attacking you. People should not look into the damage they may unleash on others, instead they should know what they are capable of doing, and in case of last resort be prepared to use the least amount of force necessary.

Law #219 - Walls are created to protect and to allow for privacy. If you build walls inside yourself, then you might be the one who is losing out. I encourage a sense of safety for everyone. I also encourage opening up some doors and seeing where they take you. There comes a point in time when those walls become damaging and are not allowing you to become the person you hope to be.

Law #220 - There are two reasons for answering a question with a question. One reason is to require the person that originally asked you a question to think for themselves as a part for their mental development. The other reason to answer with a question is to get even with them for making you think in the first place.

Law #221 - If you love someone then let them know how you feel. Time is never in abundance when you care about others. Take advantage of every opportunity to let those closest to you know how you feel. The impression you will make on them will come back to you tenfold.

Law #222 - The greatest accomplishment for this country has to be the faith we have learned to have in ourselves. The power lies in the majority pushing for the greatness of all. One person does not rule us. There are almost three hundred million people that reside in this country. Each one of those three hundred million people, one person at a time, weighs in on our greatness.

Law #223 - Has everyone not heard of the fashion police? I see styles that went out of style long ago making their attempts to return back to style. They went out for a reason, let us all move on with the times.

Law #224 - We all have different abilities and gifts in life. Some of us are meant to be writers, artists, musicians, doctors, teachers, ECT... Maybe you have not discovered what you are meant to do. Follow what inspires you and allow that to help you figure which path to take. Regardless of the outcome, it is your path as you walk down it; you are the one that creates the possibilities. Perhaps if you are unable to sketch, you are still awaiting your muse.

Law #225 - There are so many different colors in the spectrum of a rainbow. Have you noticed the brilliantly articulated stroke of nature's brush onto to the canvass of life? Life is just as colorful even to those who were born blind.

Law #226 - Knowing that you may fall to circumstance out of your control allows you the opportunity to prepare for a situation, you may be able to choose if you fall on your terms or not. As you take heed and brace yourself for the fall, there is always consolation as easy as we may fall; we all have the ability to locate the resources to climb our way back up. We just need to supply the passion essential to persevering through all of the obstacles, big or small. Know that you are never truly alone and there are those at least in thought. Some people have the resources to help, some may only able to help in spirit and to listen.

Law #227 - There is an art to the delivery of jokes. All jokes have a punch line and every story has an ending. Maybe the crowd is not ready at the time of delivery; maybe the mood has not been set. If you are willing to wait for the correct time and place, you will uncover the true gold that lies underneath the blanket of time. Sharing a light heart is the beginning of a beautiful cycle that hopefully will come back your way.

Law #228 - With the billions of people on this Earth, no one is going to please everyone all of the time. Having goodwill does not mean that you necessarily will like everyone. A common ground we should have with others is the respect for ourselves to deal with situations appropriately. Humans are by design quite flawed and apt to make mistakes. You may be willing to overlook some, while others are too deplorable, employed by evil's temptation. Until we evolve into the perfect species we must find a softer heart when dealing with troubled times may it be our own or another's.

Law #229 - Often we complicate our perception of our surroundings. Typically, the most probable answer is the correct answer. We try to speculate an adventurous saga when in fact it is normally ordinary events happening in the most inopportune and obscure times.

Law #230 - Visualizing yourself accomplishing your set goals is the first step to achieving your goals. Write a list of what you feel needs to be accomplished. If this steals the majority of your time, you may be obsessing over it. In between the

Kristin Blizzard

gray line of visualization and obsession lies ambition. A list should be simple and written to find an attainable goal.

Law #231 - The Constitution clearly states there is to be a separation between church and state. It is forbidden to have prayers in public schools; however, we allow religious beliefs to enter into politics. We have laws based on religious beliefs yet this country has been founded on the concept we all are free from religious prosecution. I do not necessarily agree with the practices of others; but, in truth, they deserve the same rights allowed to me by the first amendment. No one has the right to injure, discriminate, or harass another person based on any religious ground. I believe an older bar should not have to move simply because the new church across the street does not want to have a bar close by. As we all readily enter judgment of others, our personal beliefs are not how we should draw our conclusions, the law is meant for all of the people, not just the people that write the laws.

Law #232 - It takes an amazing person to have the character find themselves at fault, and an even more amazing person to accept responsibility and apologize for the wrong doing. With the addition of human emotion, there is typically someone in a situation that may find his or her feelings hurt. The

Murphy Didn't Know: A Second Look

truth can be painful, for this there may be sorrow for injuring the other person. We should only apologize when we truly feel sorrow for the occasion.

Law #233 - People are not meant to be toys; we cannot bend others to our will. The day may come when you will meet your match.

Law #234 - Even the toughest of people may have a very sensitive side. Often, we do stupid things in effort of hiding who we really are. There is always a way to someone's heart, we all just need to take the time and let others reveal themselves when you feel the time is right.

Law #235 - There is such a thing as having too much of a good thing. Too much ice cream, too much champagne and even too much money alters the person you are. Everything must be taken within moderation. Even the best of the best can get on your very last nerve if you never get a break from it.

Law #236 –The more I open my eyes, I realize it is not just what Murphy didn't know, a lot of us often find our crayons are not always sharpened.

Kristin Blizzard

Law #237 - Your life, just as well as my own, will lead to many new pages that have yet to be written. I cannot end this after all I have no clue as to where my future may take me. A friendly reminder for everyone is to take life in stride and try to keep an open mind as you walk down whatever path in life you choose. In the end, there is but one thing more precious than life itself: that is what we are all living for. Life is a sequence of many random events with many different possible outcomes. Life even during it's most stressful periods, is full of good times and bad times, the hard times and the easy times, the times to laugh, and the times to cry. We are a fellowship with only our best intentions and ideals to guide us as we choose from right and wrong. We can evolve into kinder and gentler people: if we do this on an individual level daily. As you carry on with your daily routines find comfort you are never alone in presence or thought, you are a mark upon the dust of time - we all are. Some people may have bigger footprints in the sand, but no one will ever be more or less important in the end than you.

Murphy Didn't Know: A Second Look

In harmony, we may find thus the glorious notes,

Each sweeter from the nectar, glorious to taste,

A simpler time, a simpler place;

A simple love, to grasp love for another.

Paradise hidden within the chasm…

A phantasmagoria so easy to shatter.

Shards reflect your beauty, please do not defy.

Both may hold beauty, yet this time is for you.

Show a million your stunning wit,

And I shall show you a million enchanted.

Allow one to witness your tenderness

Kristin Blizzard

And I will show you a million who have heard.

You have shown me, and now I believe.

You can make each day your own,

Find strength, honesty, and loyalty-

And I will show you the endless opportunities.

www.ingramcontent.com/pod-product-compliance
Lightning Source LLC
Chambersburg PA
CBHW051439280526
45785CB00003B/1347